Contents

Introduction

This Book Is for You...

> "I've learned that people will forget what you said, people will forget what you did, but people will never forget how you made them feel."
>
> UNCONFIRMED, ATTRIBUTED TO MAYA ANGELOU

To the visionary teacher, the educator, the shoelace-tier, the snack provider, the dream cultivator—this book is for you! You are the person in charge of our future's most precious commodity ... the youth of tomorrow!

No big deal, right?

We see you. The educators that are new to this. Navigating integrating the inspiration that drove you to this field with the complex realities of the education system. You already knew this work was going to be hard and you are still here, post-pandemic, after enduring one of the most challenging environments a teacher has experienced in this lifetime.

We see you. The experienced teacher who has seen many changes in education and the shifting needs of youth. The experience you have gained over the years is like no other. We'd like to see any CEO of any company trade places with a teacher like you for just one day. We wish we could give you the biggest hug you have ever felt in your life. We know you are still here because you still want to make a difference in the lives of your students.

As teachers we know you are experiencing increased social and emotional distress from your students and need as many tools as you can get to help you manage your classrooms. The intention of *Social Emotional Arts Activities for Teachers and Students to Use in the Classroom* is to support you as the teacher in your efforts to educate our children and keep them safe in ways that are easy and manageable.

It seems that a teacher's to-do list is never-ending; stacks of papers to grade, parents to contact, services to coordinate. We know on top of all of the administrative demands you have your own expectations of what it means to be the best teacher you can be. We know many teachers can be found in their downtime scrolling resources and social media platforms, searching for that perfect activity (and affordable materials!) that will ignite engagement in your classroom. Yet there is only one of you to get it all done.

We understand that you are already attending to the emotional needs of your students, and you may be wondering how you could possibly be asked to do more. Aren't there school therapists for that? Sadly, in many cases, the answer is no, or definitely not enough.

Children need support now more than ever and access to mental health resources is limited due to cost, mental health worker shortage, or cultural stigma. Especially for children that have experienced trauma, "The classroom is sometimes the most consistent and stable place in a trauma-affected student's world" (Brunzell, Stokes & Waters, 2016). You as the teacher are on the frontlines. Teachers are increasingly faced with having to help their students negotiate the stress and trauma of continued oppressive systems and global distress. A 2021 report titled *Children's Mental Health: Addressing the Impact* speaks to the urgency in finding support for young people:

> COVID-19 appears to have exacerbated and amplified what many experts call an ongoing crisis in children's mental health. Rates of adolescent suicide and self-harm were increasing even before the pandemic. Between an existing crisis in young people's mental health and COVID's impact, experts speak of a looming "tsunami" of unmet need. (Little Hoover Commission, 2021)

You have so much on your plate. We hope that this book can offer an organic and creative approach to Social Emotional Learning (SEL) objectives for your classroom. We want the information in this book to empower you and the activities to provide a sense of containment and calmness in your classroom—not just for your students but for you too! Ellen Dissanayake, a cultural anthropologist, quotes Rudolf Arnheim in her book *Homo Aestheticus* (1995) that "art, far from being a luxury, is a biologically-essential tool" (p.82). It isn't necessary to be an expert artist or have fancy art materials to help your students explore their emotional world with art. Just creating art together can offer another language that can tell us so much about those around us!

SIGNIFICANCE OF SOCIAL EMOTIONAL LEARNING IN EARLY CHILDHOOD DEVELOPMENT

Social Emotional Learning is defined by the Collaborative for Academic, Social, and Emotional Learning (CASEL) as, "The process through which children and adults understand and manage emotions, set and achieve positive goals, feel and show empathy for others, establish and maintain positive relationships, and make responsible decisions" (CASEL, 2024). These skill development areas include a wide variety of interpersonal and social skills that holistically benefit the child across a lifetime and into adulthood. SEL concepts include five core competencies: self-awareness, self-management, social awareness, relationship skills and responsible decision-making. There is a substantial amount of research that indicates that there is a significant correlation between academic performance and social and emotional skills, and that early social and emotional competency can lay a foundation for healthy development across the lifespan. Additionally, practicing social and emotional skills can provide early intervention that has been shown to reduce negative and antisocial behavior such as criminal violence and drug use, and increase protective factors for later mental health difficulties (Wigelsworth *et al.*, 2022).

Social Emotional Learning is a really effective strategy that is very much in alignment with a trauma-informed model. A trauma-informed model provides helpful experiences for *all* your students, not just those that may have experienced trauma. Trauma-informed care is about establishing a framework to recognize and respond to the effects of trauma. There are different types of trauma, including acute trauma: a trauma that is short-lived (natural disaster), and complex trauma: trauma that occurs repeatedly over a long period of time (physical or sexual abuse). Trauma-informed care focuses on the physical and emotional safety of the teacher and the youth (see Bath, 2015). Trauma-informed strategies offer a sense of empowerment and control that can counteract the feelings of stress, anxiety, doubt and fear that may result from trauma. Many SEL competencies, such as self-awareness and self-management, help children that have been impacted by trauma and adversity mitigate some of the distress that they might suffer from. Learning how to identify and articulate how you feel and what you might need can really empower these children and *all* children.

HOW THE ARTS CAN SUPPORT SOCIAL EMOTIONAL LEARNING

So now that we know that SEL is vital for every child's development, let's talk about how to implement it in ways that are easy and engaging for both your students and for you! The arts offer countless opportunities to address SEL; visual art, dance, music, theater are all wonderful vehicles for building self-awareness and deepening relationships resulting in a happier, more regulated little person. Because we, the authors of this book, are both art therapists and use visual art as our approach, the information and activities given here will be focused on this discipline.

Have you ever heard of art therapy? Art therapy is facilitated by credentialed mental health professionals with master's level or higher degrees and uses art media, the creative process and the resulting artwork as a therapeutic and healing process. Clients, young, old and in-between, are able to explore their feelings, reconcile emotional conflicts, foster self-awareness, manage behavior, develop social skills, improve reality orientation, reduce anxiety and increase self-esteem (ATCB, 2024). What doesn't art therapy do?! As art therapists, we have worked in a variety of community settings and have witnessed first-hand the power of art-based approaches to social emotional learning. That being said, don't worry: you won't be practicing art therapy, but what you *can* do is use the art-making process to enhance social and emotional skill development.

We want to take a quick moment here to emphasize that you do not need to be skilled in visual art to provide visual art-based SEL exercises. Repeat after me, I do not need to be skilled in visual art to provide visual art-based SEL exercises. And that goes for your students as well. All too many times we hear from teachers that they don't feel artistic enough to implement art-based exercises with their students. Students will benefit regardless of skill level. Promise.

Now that we've got that out of the way, let's consider how visual art can provide lots of opportunities for SEL. The act of conceptualizing, exploring, creating, reflecting and sharing our artwork has been shown to really help children (and adults!). At a very basic level, when kids are making art they are engaging in a sensory experience that has been shown to **increase emotional regulation**. As you probably know, emotional regulation is the ability to monitor and modulate your emotional experiences. We think of this kind of like a thermostat—if it's too cold the heat turns on and if it's too hot the air conditioning turns on. Emotional regulation is a skill we learn to help us manage all the ups and downs of our emotions in ways that are appropriate to context. Using bright colors to color in shapes, moving paint across the paper, or exploring the softness of modeling clay can help kids regulate by getting out of their heads and into their bodies. Making art can help kids become or stay calm. When kids are calm, they will be more likely to take in new information which is helpful both socially, emotionally and academically. Being able to emotionally regulate has significant advantages in all stages of life but specific to childhood, being able to regulate increases a student's feelings of competency, which leads to another benefit of art-making and SEL!

Making art has been shown to **increase a young person's self-esteem**. Expressing one's self and being seen and heard by others in that expression can feel very affirming and thus can build a child's self-confidence. When we feel confident in ourselves, we are more likely to take positive risks (risks that are more likely to have positive outcomes like raising our hands in class, introducing ourselves to a new friend). Creating art also takes a great amount of problem-solving. Moving an idea from inside your head to a piece of paper or sculpture will take planning, organizing and most likely an ability to navigate through several attempts!

Lastly (although we could go on and on about the benefits of art in SEL!), creating, reflecting and sharing our art **builds communication skills and increases empathy**. When students create art alongside their peers, they engage in both a verbal and visual dialogue. Seeing a person's art can deepen understanding of another person's experience. When students have positive communication with their peers, can give and receive empathy and manage conflict more effectively, they can enjoy school more!

In order to help you integrate art and SEL in ways that are developmentally appropriate, we've summarized some theoretical information into a handy table that presents children's development, common challenges, potential reasons for challenges, social emotional needs and ways to address developmental social emotional needs with art.

ART-BASED SOCIAL EMOTIONAL STRATEGIES FOR POSITIVE DEVELOPMENT

Age: 5 years old

Developmental markers

- Increased independence, curiosity and a growing sense of self
- Still learning to regulate their emotions and behavior

Common challenging behavior

- Temper tantrums
- Defiance
- Whining
- Exaggerating needs
- Possessiveness
- Taking things and lying about it
- Exclusion
- Hitting, pushing, biting
- Restlessness or clumsiness
- Bossiness
- Separation anxiety
- Competitiveness

What's happening?

- Increased brain development may cause difficulty with motor skills that once came easily, causing frustration
- Increased brain development allows for more awareness of inconsistencies in academics, causing frustration
- Social skills are developing and friends are becoming important factors, yet children base preference on shared play interests and prefer smaller groups

- Experiencing increase in cognitive capacity and developing an ability to understand that others might have a different experience, yet still struggling with inner moral conflict

Social Emotional Need

- Clear and consistent boundaries, expectations and appropriate consequences
- Positive reinforcement and encouragement for resilient behavior
- Practice problem-solving skills
- Opportunities to express emotion in constructive ways
- Modeling of appropriate social and emotional responses

Art response

- Art materials that provide a variety of kinesthetic experiences
- Art materials that explore color and high contrast (dark color on light colored paper)
- Free draw on large paper with less structured materials i.e. paint sticks, pastel
- Using found objects or recyclables to create, i.e. creating structures with cardboard and tape
- Exploration and play with materials. i.e. using modeling clay and figurines

Age: 6 years old

Developmental markers

- Increased fine motor skills
- Adopting socially constructed gender-specific behavior
- Increase in cognitive capacities, moving from concrete thought to abstract thought
- Increased verbal capacities

Common challenging behavior

- Crying and whining
- Tantrums, hitting, kicking
- Indecision
- Sensitive to criticism
- Difficulty sitting still
- Avoidance to playing with the opposite sex
- Learned helplessness "can't do it" attitude
- Lie or cheat to win games
- Stubborn determinism
- Eager for approval, difficulty taking blame

What's happening?

- Increased brain development, dopamine levels increase and allow for a greater sense of focus and self-control
- Moving from concrete to abstract and symbolic thinking
- Increased ability to hold attention for 20–30 mins

- Beginning to develop self-evaluation and becoming more aware of self in relation to others can impact child's ability to admit fault or apologize

Social Emotional Need

- Need for routine and ritual to create a feeling of security
- Encouragement and support to persist and problem solve during moments of frustration to help with development of a positive self-concept

Art response

- Free drawing/painting on larger paper (i.e. 12x18 for drawing, 18x24 for painting)
- Introduce and explore subject matter that is meaningful to child from their immediate environments
- Place emphasis on exploration of material vs. final product
- Creating visual patterns
- Provide choice (2–3 max) in material and content and provide time for children to develop mastery before changing material
- Soft air-dry clay
- Tempera paint in a variety of colors: primary and secondary
- Avoid instantaneous art projects

Age: 7 years old

Developmental markers

- Advancement in cognitive capacities: logical and linear processes, reciprocity, reversibility, conservation
- Able to develop true empathy
- Trying to build their own identities through task mastery, internal processing and comparison to others
- Increased self-control
- Gender identity

Common challenging behavior

- Withdrawn
- Perfectionistic
- Difficulty transitioning from task to task
- Becomes frustrated if not given time to finish a task
- Overly dramatic "I might as well die"
- Sensitive to rejection
- View life as unfair
- Easily disappointed
- Develop fears that were not present earlier

What's happening?

- Environment is increasingly playing a role in development
- Continued increase in dopamine levels makes planning and focusing easier and may make it hard to stop
- High self-imposed standards due to cognitive capacities that increase self-awareness and comparison
- Increased self-awareness and abilities for self-management can lead to quick fatigue
- Increase in empathy and perspective, taking leads to less egocentric and more social play, adhering to rules vs. cheating to win

Social Emotional Need

- Developing confidence in self through task mastery
- Needs ample time to work through projects
- Access to privacy with regards to their bodies
- Reminders to take breaks
- Opportunities to engage in unstructured social time
- Opportunities to engage in perspective-taking activities

Art response

- Multi-step art projects
- Soft lead graphite pencils and ability to erase or redo
- Structured art projects, i.e. art about a concept vs. free choice
- Provide choice (2-3 max) in material and content and provide time for children to develop mastery before changing material
- Soft air-dry clay
- Tempera paint in a variety of colors: primary, secondary, tertiary
- Collaborative art, i.e. team projects, individual projects that form a group project
- Arts and science integration
- Problem solving art (i.e. build a bridge with only string and straws)
- Perspective taking in art (draw from the perspective of a dog, a friend, a parent, etc.)
- Avoid stereotyped projects that may lead to predictable results

Age: 8 years old

Developmental markers

- Tends to be outgoing
- Has high energy levels
- Enjoys school
- Increase in fine motor skills
- Independence in hygiene activities
- Curious about sexuality
- "Decentration": the ability to focus on several features of a task at a time

Common challenging behavior

- Rushes through projects
- Excessive self-criticism
- Increased focus on peer relationships
- Testing limits
- Mood swings

What's happening?

- Brain development increases abilities for long-term memory
- Beginning of hormonal development

Social Emotional Need

- Opportunities for physical energy release
- Simple directions
- Opportunities for hands-on exploration
- Ample time to add details

Art response

- Art activities that advance in need for fine motor skills, e.g. drawing, sewing, beading, sculpting
- Multi-step art projects
- Collaborative projects: posters, models
- Provide a wide range of open-ended topics for differing student interests especially with regards to gender
- Show acceptance of any student-initiated subject matter
- Support the development of meaningful, exciting and intense involvement in personal self-expression
- Materials that are structured enough to provide student with expression and mastery: soft lead pencils, chalk, pastels, tempera paint

Age: 9 years old

Developmental markers

- Able to express thoughts and feelings to others
- Persistent
- Increased independence
- Highs and lows in physical activity
- May show early signs of puberty
- Starts to show less interest in primary caregivers
- Meaningful relationships with friends
- Understands romantic relationships but has little interest in them

Common challenging behavior

- May worry more
- Tends to be sensitive and get feelings hurt more easily
- Puts more pressure on academic performance
- Avoidance of situations where they feel they might fail
- Desires more privacy and is more conscious of their body
- Has multiple somatic complaints in response to challenging tasks
- Roughhousing

What's happening?

- Brain development allows for pleasure in mastering new tasks as well as a decrease in impulsive behaviors, i.e. outbursts.
- Increasing awareness of the world around them and a desire to produce realistic representations
- Desire for societal approval

Social Emotional Need

- Outlets for physical play in safe ways, i.e. team sports
- Intellectual tasks that build self-confidence and mastery
- Opportunities to engage in independent tasks
- Identifying and practicing coping skills for managing anxiety
- Practicing compassion and self-compassion

Art response

- Support independent decisions about content of art and encourage expression of unique identities
- Provide a variety of expressive materials (drawing, painting, sculpting, collage, found objects, photography, etc.) to encourage exploration and mastery of a new material
- Include other methods of expression that are *not* drawing, i.e. collage, printmaking, photography
- Provide ample time for incorporation of details
- Collaborative projects; murals, dioramas
- Planning and problem solving in art
- Art about different feeling states; masks, color exploration
- Encourage exploration in materials but also provide opportunity for student to create a product they find meaningful

Age: 10 years old

Developmental markers

- Increased concentration, attention span and ability to regulate emotions
- Concrete and logical
- Desire to organize and classify
- Increased fine/gross motor skills, balance, agility, speed
- Strong sense of right and wrong
- Easy going and confident
- Social relationships and peer groups increase in their importance
- Growing sense of cultural identity
- Pubescent changes

Common challenging behavior

- Excessive concern with belonging to the group
- Spending excessive time maneuvering through social interactions
- Quick to anger

What's happening?

- Brain development in the prefrontal cortex allows for advancements in cognitive processes such as problem solving, memory, impulse control, consciousness and movement
- Brain development in the right hemisphere responsible for emotions and spatial reasoning
- Welfare is associated with that of the group; belonging to an identified group creates a sense of security
- Adapting emotional responses to be more socially acceptable
- Moving towards social perspective-taking

Social Emotional Need

- Modeling positive communication and relationship skills
- Practice with conflict resolution skills
- Provide opportunities for group and social activities
- Support from meaningful social relationships

Art response

- Cultural exploration of self and other
- Storytelling in art: masks, comic strips, puppets.
- Variety of expressive art making that include other forms of art-making other than drawing: printmaking, collage, photography, assemblage, clay, mosaics

SOURCES: GREGORY (2002) AND RAY (2016)

HOW TO USE THIS BOOK

As a source of structure for the activities or "recipes" in this book, we use the well-researched and evidence-based framework created by The Collaborative for Academic, Social, and Emotional Learning (CASEL). Many states across the U.S. have begun to adapt and integrate these Social Emotional Learning skills into classroom curricula, which offer us a shared language to come back to. As you explore the art recipes you will see that the activities are separated into five competency areas identified by CASEL (2022):

- Self-awareness
- Self-management
- Social awareness
- Relationship skills
- Responsible decision-making.

We like to think of these five social emotional learning competencies as ingredients in a cake—each can stand alone but when mixed together they create something delicious!

You can flip through each of the five skill development areas to learn more about what these categories mean, why they are significant to a child's development, how the art process can create opportunities to develop each competency, and tips to help things run smoothly. You can also just start from the beginning and slowly work your way through the book! We have taken care to be intentional with the way the recipes are organized so that students are scaffolded in their SEL skill development as they move through the book. Not all recipes as they are written will be appropriate for ALL developmental levels. Refer back to the SEL and Development Table earlier in this chapter if you have questions about whether an activity will be suitable for your age group. Also, you are the expert on your students! Feel free to use the recipes as a jumping off point and modify as you see fit.

The five competency areas are not just for your students. As with all of the SEL categories you are in the perfect position to model what this looks like for your students. Every teacher has experienced the moment when your plans just don't work out due to an emotional outburst from one of your students. We hope that the definitions and applicable skills you will read about in each section can help you just as much as the students. We often instruct the grown-ups to make their own art right along with the kiddos so that you can use the opportunity for modeling, mirroring and bonding through shared experience.

Social Emotional Learning with Art

A recipe for connection!

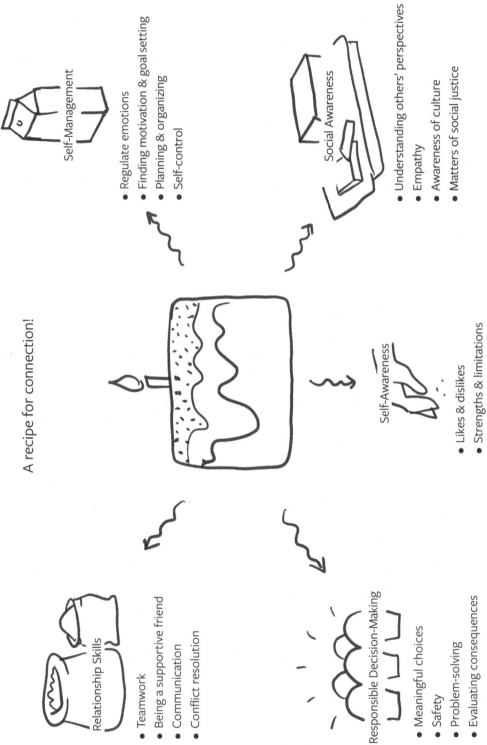

Self-Management
- Regulate emotions
- Finding motivation & goal setting
- Planning & organizing
- Self-control

Social Awareness
- Understanding others' perspectives
- Empathy
- Awareness of culture
- Matters of social justice

Self-Awareness
- Likes & dislikes
- Strengths & limitations
- Emotions
- Awareness of thoughts

Relationship Skills
- Teamwork
- Being a supportive friend
- Communication
- Conflict resolution

Responsible Decision-Making
- Meaningful choices
- Safety
- Problem-solving
- Evaluating consequences

HOW TO USE THE ART RECIPES

There are many ways you can utilize the art recipes. First, you can use the recipes much like you would use a regular recipe in a cookbook. Recipes are often used as a starting point for inspiration. You can take a little here, add some spice there or change things up as you see fit to curate a "menu" to meet the specific needs of your students. You can also follow the recipes exactly as they are laid out or change the "ingredients" to match the materials you have available. You can offer a recipe to your whole class, or you can give a prompt to a smaller group of students. Let's say you have noticed that your classroom could use some support in developing and keeping relationships or perhaps you notice a need for more self-management to create a calmer learning environment. Flip to the SEL category that can best support this goal.

As the heartbeat of the classroom, you know your students better than anyone and you are in a great position to assess their needs. In fact, art activities such as these are great assessment tools to get to know your students better. It may offer you a little window into their emotional worlds. Perhaps you will not have time (or it may be out of your scope of practice) to address the needs of your students yourself, but using the information you learn during an art activity can be useful when making referrals to other resources available at your school.

Second, you may choose to use the recipes as an integrated part of your school day. This can be done by carving out 15 to 20 minutes so that art and SEL becomes a part of your daily routine. It can be very difficult to do so, but we recommend this option. From a trauma-informed approach, as you know, engaging your students in routines that are consistent and predictable can really help lessen anxiety.

TIPS FOR CLASSROOM INTEGRATION OF ART RECIPES

At whichever level you decide to implement the art recipe activities into your classroom we have gathered a lot of tips from our past experiences that we would love to share with you!

First and foremost, we encourage you as the facilitator to *stay curious*. The art recipes have steps and guidelines; however, the outcome of each activity will look different for every student. It's important to practice cultural humility and keep your mind open when a student represents something that looks different to what you expected. The recipes are intended to have an element of free expression and even though we provide you with examples of student artwork, keep in mind that each student's work will look completely unique. That's a great thing, and when you celebrate this in your classroom you encourage diversity and individuality.

Setting the stage

The first tip we have might seem a little obvious, but we still think it's important to note. "Setting the stage," as famed art educator and art therapist Judith Rubin (1978) stated, is about knowing the environment. Setting the stage considers the organization of the space and presentation, distribution and clean-up of materials, and the interests and energy levels of your students. Other questions to consider ahead of time might include:

- Is there adequate lighting?
- How are the tables organized? Single desks? Groups of desks?
- How are the tables covered for the art process?
- Is there adequate space and access to materials?
- Is there a place/materials to clean messes? Garbage cans? Sink?
- Is there a space to store unfinished and/or completed projects?

Art materials

Art materials are wonderful ways to engage your students' behaviors and interactions. Different art mediums have different qualities inherent to that material. For example, drawing with pencils and stencils is a very different experience to molding clay. Pencils and stencils are very structured and will tend to elicit a very focused behavior from participants, whereas modeling clay is more explorative and tactile, which tends to increase self-expression.

Experimenting with materials before the workshops will give you insight and empathy for your students and how they might react when they are engaging with the materials. Being mindful of how materials will influence the relationships between your students before beginning is an important part of setting the stage for success.

Whenever possible, offering some choice in materials will provide developmentally appropriate autonomy and confidence. For example, younger children may become frustrated when using materials that require detail-oriented, fine motor skills, i.e. tying, twisting, some types of sculpting. Being mindful of the capabilities of your participants and offering choice or multiple "access points" will ensure that your participants feel able to meet the expectations of the project.

Lastly, making sure that art materials are inclusive is *very* important when providing art projects in the classroom. Making sure that you have ethnically considerate color palettes and imagery that represents a wide variety of bodies and body types is an absolute *must*!

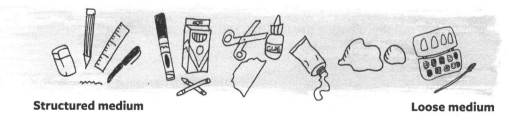

Structured medium   **Loose medium**

Talking about the art

As mentioned earlier, encouraging little people to share what they made is a great way to build self-esteem, communicate and increase empathy. When a child asks, "Do you like it?" it can be hard not to say "Yes! Of course! It's *sooo* amazing!" Most kids love praise and seek affirmation from one of their favorite people—you! Although important to hear praise and affirmation from trusted adults, focusing the discussion about the art to come from the perspective of the creator is a great way to help children to develop self-competency. Practice using and modeling non-value-based dialogue like, "I'm wondering...," "Could you tell me more about...," "Is there a story about..."

Additionally, art-making is a wonderful time to "catch" a student engaging in positive social and emotional behaviors. As students are creating, comment on the positive behaviors you see them engaging in independently or socially: "Wow, you are really focusing," or "I noticed how the two of you have really figured out how to share those materials" or "I just wanted to let you know that I watched you work through some frustration by taking a deep breath."

Working with mistakes...

If you have your students create art in your classroom, you have likely heard some version of, "Teacher, I made a mistake! I need a new piece of paper!" This is a sign that there is likely a critical self-judgment about their abilities and it's an opportunity to shift the child towards working through mistakes. Try to keep your energy calm and positive. If frustration arises, acknowledge the artist's desires for perfection with gentleness while opening the door for turning the "mistake" into a "happy accident" or opportunity to problem solve. If a child exclaims that they don't like their drawing, you can respond with "Don't like it *yet*!" Helping your students to identify what exactly they don't like about their art and possible ways to change it is also a good way to help children develop resilience. As you read through the chapters, we will try to highlight how these tips might apply to the art process in relation to the five SEL competencies.

Take a look at the following figures. The Iceberg shows different types of challenging behaviors you might observe in your classroom as well as the underlying SEL need. Lastly, we provide a graphic on supporting your students that shows common phrases you might hear from students and how you can respond.

The Iceberg

Keeping your cool during art making time isn't easy when there are many behaviors that can heat up our frustration. There is typically an underlying vulnerability to outward behavior and when we connect with the emotion underneath the iceberg we can keep our "empathy brain" alert and ready.

CRITICAL OF ART WITH SELF AND OTHERS, WILL NOT STOP WHEN IT'S TIME TO STOP

ASKING FOR APPROVAL AFTER EVERY STEP

THROWING MATERIALS

FIDGETY, DROPPING THINGS FREQUENTLY, DISRUPTING OTHERS

NOT FOLLOWING THE DIRECTION OR REFUSING THE ACTIVITY

PERCEIVED NEGATIVE BEHAVIOR

VULNERABLE EMOTIONS TO ADDRESS

Shy
Unworthy
Uncertain
Fearful
Left-out
Nervous
Emotional
Incapable
Overwhelmed
Embarrassed
Sensory sensitivity
Judged
Over-stimulated
Tired

SELF-CRITICISM, DOUBT AND SHAME

- Consider classroom mantra or cheer around turning mistakes into happy accidents.
- Everyone can join in with frequent time reminders.
- Create a safe space in your room for unfinished work. It can be a work in progress!

MEASURING UP TO OTHERS AND SEEING THEMSELVES AS BAD IN COMPARISON

- A child might be seeking your approval because they feel less than what they see around the room.
- Noticing and praising a unique detail of their work can be useful. Name that we grow when something is challenging.

DYSREGULATION IN THE BODY

- Consider a quick grounding break for all students, e.g., a big breath.
- If possible, have a box that allows each child to have their own art materials.
- Routine is key, consider if your activity time is predictable and structured for the student.

FEELING FORCED AND/OR A LACK OF CONFIDENCE

- If a child is still making art, encourage it.
- It can be very helpful to name what might be happening for kiddo, e.g., "I notice you are not feeling the activity for today and that's OK, I wonder what else you could make."

Supporting your students

There are common phrases you might hear while making art with youth. Here are some considerations on how to validate concerns while getting your students back on a growth mindset for learning.

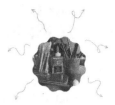

"Teacher, do you like it?"
FOR THE KID WHO WANTS YOUR CONSTANT APPROVAL:

- Point out something specific you notice, e.g. "I see all the great colors! How did you do that?"
- Refer to all those great sentence starters to help students reflect on the process, e.g. "I notice how you..."
- Redirect and ask student to share their observations, e.g. "What do you see? Do you have a favorite part. Can you show me?"

"I can't/or I don't like it."
FOR THE KID WHO IS VERY CRITICAL OF THEMSELVES

- When a child says "I don't like it," consider the response, "Don't like it yet!"
- Encourage them to start drawing and see what happens.
- Use the phrase, "This is just take one; let's see what take two will bring."

"Teacher, I'm done."
FOR THE KID WHO FINISHES TOO EARLY

- Share an observation about an area of their work, remind the student you can add layers to get even more meaning in the process.
- Perhaps the kiddo needs a little break. Encourage your student to take a drink of water or walk away for a short moment and come back.
- Have some scratch paper on back up for free drawing.

"I'm not good at that."
FOR THE KID WHO MIGHT FEEL AFRAID TO TAKE RISKS

- The students might be getting overwhelmed; try breaking the instruction into small bites.
- Offer a brainstorming session using materials that are not permanent in nature, e.g. dry erase board, sticky notes, scratch paper or pencil and eraser.
- Ask the kiddo to come up with a mantra to repeat to themselves. If they can't think of one, see if a classmate can help them out.

"What are we supposed to do?"
FOR THE KID WHO STRUGGLES WITH FOCUS

- Invite the student to join you in explaining the project steps to boost confidence and encourage participation.
- Offer several entry points for learning, e.g. show an example of an art piece that you made ahead of time.
- Provide written steps on the board if possible.
- Prompt student to observe what others are doing.

"Will you draw me a...?"
FOR THE KID WHO WANTS YOU TO DO IT FOR THEM

- Resist the urge to draw the image for them as it might cause them to feel incapable and discouraged.
- Consider responding with, "Let's both draw."
- Grab a separate piece of paper and support the student by asking them to scribble along with you. Let's say the child would like support with drawing a circle, together you can make the circular shapes that will help the child do it all on her own.

SUGGESTED OUTLINE FOR A RECIPE SESSION (SEL ART ACTIVITY TIME)

As noted earlier, predictable routines help you in creating a classroom environment that values social emotional learning and that is trauma informed. Take a look at this suggested outline for implementing the arts and SEL recipes in your classroom.

- Grounding exercise (2–3 minutes)
  - We recommend a grounding exercise of your choice. Examples might be a big group stretch or a brief breathing exercise.
- Introduce the topic (2–3 minutes)
  - Introduce the topic of the day by reading the title and the description of the exercise along with questions to consider while engaged in the art making process. During this time, you can generate examples from the students with examples that are relevant to them in their lives.
- Art-making time (20 minutes)
  - Students explore the theme with art-making. Extra points for participating with the students. Remind students (and yourself!) that it is about the process and not all about the product.
- Share and clean up (5 minutes)
  - Some students might like to share; others not so much. We recommend offering the students the choice to share if they would like to. If time runs over, you can always have them share with the person next to them. Older students might prefer this. On each activity we have offered you big picture questions to get the kids considering how the activity encourages the SEL category. Depending on age, you might adjust vocabulary and tone of voice.

Ok! Are you ready to get going? You've got this!

Chapter 1

SELF-AWARENESS

"My art piece means that you should be yourself because 'you are enough just as you are.' No one should be ashamed or feel less than anyone else, we are all human and we all have flaws but those are what make us human. I chose these bright colors because they *pop* and they stand out. With these colors I am saying it's ok to be different and you don't always have to blend in."

MIDDLE SCHOOL STUDENT

The quote above highlights how the art process helped this student explore and name her unique point of view. The artist uses words grounded in self-validation and compassion to describe her work. There is also a sense of how she connected her feelings to how other people her age feel. We can see that it was the art that brought her to this wonderful conclusion that it's great to stand out! One can imagine how this concept might stay with her the next time she is feeling left out, criticized or overwhelmed.

Self-awareness helps students know themselves. When we have self-awareness, we are better able to express how we feel and ask for what we need. Self-awareness can also look like helping students make connections between the feeling they experience and how it shows up as sensations in the body. This might look like a student drawing butterflies over the stomach to represent anxiety. If we are able to name our experience, it helps us communicate to others our needs and sets the stage for better self-care.

Consider what early intervention and education can do on the journey towards knowing yourself and your needs. As therapists, we see many adults in our practice that are just now learning helpful strategies to better understand their emotions. Perhaps you can relate. This is because many patterns of thinking become ingrained by the time we are out of school. When we think of it that way, doesn't it seem necessary that we offer self-awareness strategies early? Helping your students learn more about their thoughts and feelings now will set them up for greater awareness as they grow.

Art can offer a multitude of ways to explore identity and self-concepts. It doesn't always take the form of a self-portrait. In art therapy we often say that there are no accidents. This statement means that even though we are making art about another person, symbol or shape, we are in some ways expressing something about ourselves. When you start to pay attention to how children describe their art you will begin to hear little bits about their point of view. It's not always easy to describe how we think and feel, especially for a child. Art gives us the opportunity to turn our inward thoughts outward so that we may describe our inner world to others. It helps us name strengths and limitations and offers the time necessary to sit with thoughts and feelings so that we can understand them better.

Using the art process can help you assess what's happening in your classrooms. It will help you gain awareness towards cultural beliefs offering you helpful ways to engage your students in matters important to them. If you follow the facilitator tip to remain curious with an open mind, you will model the same for your students where students can feel seen and heard in the space. Butterflies drawn over the stomach or creating feeling monsters for example, is a great way to get youth talking about anxiety ... a topic children often do not have the language for.

MIND MAP

Mindfulness is a skill that helps us focus on the present moment. When we practice mindfulness, we can calm our minds and build our self-awareness about how we are thinking and feeling, and what we might be needing. Have you ever practiced being mindful? What types of things do you do to be mindful?

Materials:

- Journal or paper
- Drawing tools (crayons, colored pencils and/or markers)

Steps:

1. Close your eyes or find somewhere to softly gaze and take three big deep breaths.
2. Place a drawing tool on your paper. Without lifting it, take a deep breath in, pausing at the top of your breath. Slowly exhale and move your drawing tool in any direction that feels pleasing for you.
3. Continue to move your drawing tool in different directions as you breathe in and out.
4. Continue for five big breaths.
5. Use drawing tools to create lines, shapes and colors to represent how you feel in your body. You can fill in the space with words and/or colors that express how you feel.

Big picture questions:

1. How did this activity make you feel today?
2. I wonder if we were to make one later today, or tomorrow, do you think your mind map might look different? How so?
3. Do you notice any similarities with other students today?
4. When might be a good time to make another mind map on your own? Why is that?

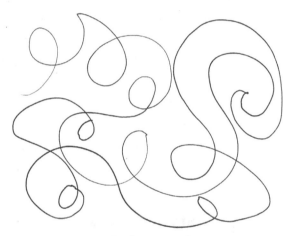

Student example

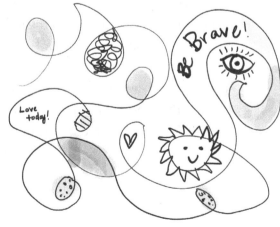

Student example

MOOD METER

Our emotions come in so many shapes and sizes! Practice self-awareness by creating a tool that helps you to identify how you are feeling. We all tend to feel the following four emotional states at some point: angry, excited, sad and calm. Can you think of a time you experienced one of these emotions?

Materials:

- Journal or paper drawing tools (crayons, colored pencils and/or markers)
- Watercolor paint palette, brushes, water (Optional: watercolor paper)

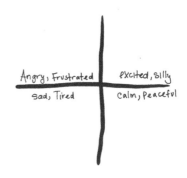

Steps:

1. Start by drawing a cross in your journal.
2. Label each section with a different feeling state.
3. What colors, shapes, lines or symbols come to mind when you think of each feeling state?
4. Use drawing tools and/or watercolor paints to create lines, shapes and colors that represent each feeling state to you.
5. After you are done, consider how you are feeling and point to an area on your mood meter.

Big picture questions:

1. Sometimes kids think that we shouldn't feel sad or angry, but it's a necessary emotion we all experience! Which emotion of the mood meter is the most unpleasant for you? How about the emotion that is most pleasant for you?
2. Do you think your mood meter could help you share with others how you feel? Why?
3. When might be a good time to use your mood meter?

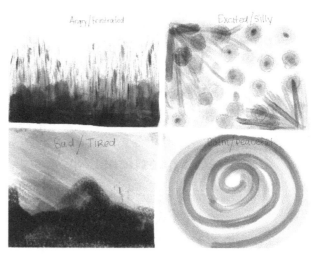

Student example

28

MOODY LITTLE CREATURES

Now that you have your mood meter we can use it in a lot of different creative ways. For this activity, use your imagination to create a creature that can help you tell different stories about your emotions and feelings.

Materials:

- Journal or paper
- Drawing tools (crayons, colored pencils and/or markers)
- Ripped or torn paper works great too

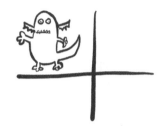

Steps:

1. Start by drawing a cross in your journal just like you did for your mood meter.
2. Label each section with the same feeling state as your mood meter.
3. Make a little creature for each square.
4. Use drawing tools to think about how this little creature expresses how they are feeling. Maybe with how they hold their body, or the expression on their face.
5. When you are done, make up a story about each little creature. Where do they live? Are they friends? What types of things do they like to do together? See where your imagination takes you.

Big picture questions:

1. Have you ever felt so angry that you felt like a monster?
2. It's OK to feel angry, everyone does. What are examples of healthy ways to express our anger?
3. Great job with your little creatures, what might happen if your calm creature spoke to your angry creature? It's fun to think about the ways they might interact. Draw a picture and talk about it.

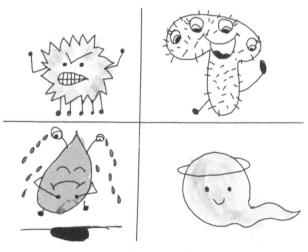

Student example

VISUAL BODY SCAN

Our body is a great tool that can help us recognize when we are having an emotion or feeling. Paying attention to how we feel in our body is an awesome skill that can help give us clues to how we might continue a feeling or work towards changing a feeling! Sometimes it can be hard to sit with feelings in our bodies—make sure you listen to your body and if you start to feel nervous or scared know that you can stop and draw something else.

Materials:

 Journal or paper
- Drawing tools (crayons, colored pencils and/or markers)

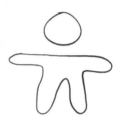

Steps:

1. Start by creating a simple outline of a body.
2. Close your eyes or find somewhere to gaze and take three big deep breaths.
3. Starting at either the top of your head or the bottom of your feet, slowly focus on how you feel in each area of your body.
4. Use drawing tools to create lines, shapes and colors to represent how you feel in your body.

Big picture questions:

1. What are some of the ways your body tells you when you are feeling excited, happy and joyful?
2. What are some of the ways your body tells you when you are feeling nervous, anxious or afraid?
3. What are some of the ways your body tells you when you are feeling calm?
4. When we have so many things happening around us, how do you think we can listen better to our bodies?
5. Have you figured out a way to calm your body when it's feeling excited?

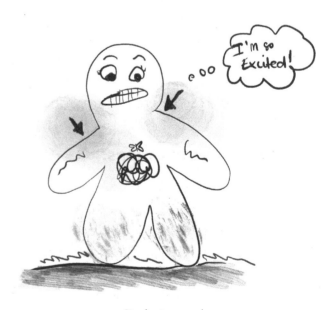

Student example

RAINBOW MINDFULNESS

Sometimes when there is a lot going on it can be really helpful to pause and practice the skill of mindfulness by noticing our surroundings. In this exercise you will be practicing mindfulness and self-awareness by noticing all the different colors of the rainbow that are around you! When you pause to notice and name what is around you, you might notice something new that has actually been there all along! Do you see anything new?

Materials:

- Journal or paper
- Drawing tools (crayons, colored pencils and/or markers)

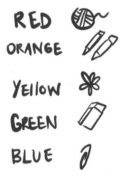

Steps:

1. Start by taking a big belly breath.
2. Quietly bring your awareness to the room around you.
3. Start to look around the room and find things that are all the colors of the rainbow. ROY-G-BIV! Red, orange, yellow, green, blue, indigo, violet.
4. Use a page in your journal to draw something you can see of each color of the rainbow. If you can't see something of every color, use your imagination!

Big picture questions:

1. Why is it helpful to slow down and notice what is around you?
2. Did anyone notice something in the classroom that they have never noticed before?
3. If you were feeling really distracted at school, do you think this exercise would be helpful? Why?

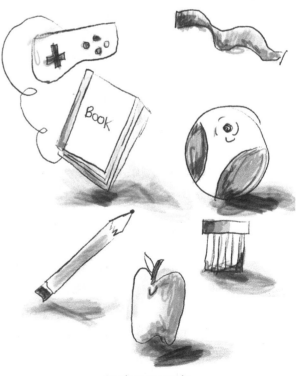

Student example

PAY ATTENTION TO YOUR THOUGHTS

Thoughts are ideas, memories and opinions that pop up into our awareness at any given time. Scientists say that we have at least one thought every two seconds. That's a lot of thoughts per day! We are always thinking even if we aren't paying attention to our thoughts. Let's practice some awareness of thoughts by drawing thought bubbles to practice paying attention. Draw words or images to represent some of your thoughts.

Materials:

- Journal or paper
- Drawing tools (crayons, colored pencils and/or markers)

Steps:

1. Let's start the practice of paying attention to our thoughts by filling the page up with thought bubbles that we can use to draw or write in.
2. Now the fun begins, start to draw or write your thoughts as they pop into your head.
3. Have fun! There is absolutely no wrong way to do this exercise. Our thoughts can sometimes be all over the place. One moment we are thinking about soccer and the next we are thinking about bananas.
4. When you are finished, have a look at where your thinking took you today.

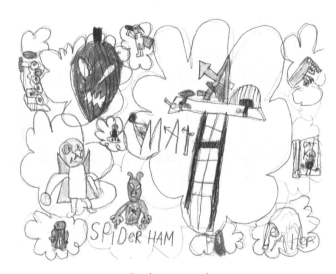

Student example

Big picture questions:

1. Why is it helpful to think about our thoughts and practice paying attention to them?
2. Did anyone notice you were thinking about something earlier in the day, or wondering what will happen later?
3. Our thoughts are like that a lot of the time and sometimes it's helpful to notice our thoughts as they arise. Can you guess why? Is there a time when you think it could be helpful to try this drawing activity? Why?

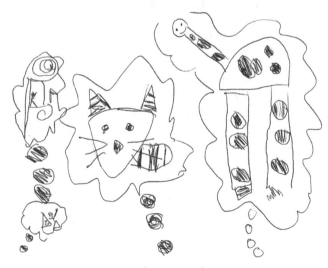

Student example

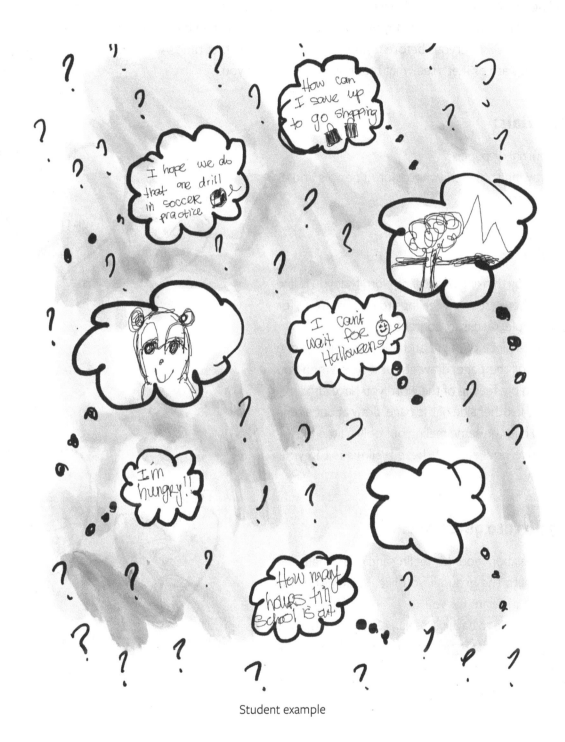

Student example

FEELINGS COME IN ALL SIZES!

Feelings come in many sizes. Have you ever noticed that some feelings show up in a big way while some feelings show up just a tiny bit? For example, you could feel BIG nervous before riding a roller coaster but small nervous before trying a new food for the first time. All feelings are part of life, and all feelings are ok. Let's see what that might look like for you.

Materials:

- Journal or paper
- Drawing tools (crayons, colored pencils and/or markers)

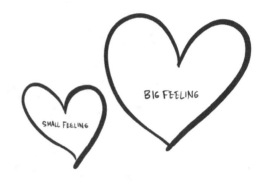

Steps:

1. Start by thinking of a feeling word that you relate to. There are many feelings to choose from, for example, mad, sad, content or loved.
2. Take a piece of paper and fold it in half. On one side of the page, draw about a time when you had a big feeling of the word you have chosen.
3. On the other side of the page, draw about a time you had the same feeling but only a little bit.
4. Notice how each of these feelings felt in your body.

Big picture questions:

1. Share about your big feeling and your small feeling with the group if you like. Which one was more pleasant for you?
2. Is it wrong to have big feelings? Why or why not?
3. If you were having a big feeling, what do you think is the best way to share it with others?

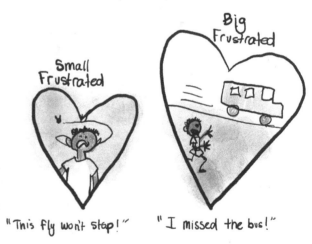

Student example

FEELINGS COME IN MANY WAYS

Feelings come in many different ways. Remember when you explored how feelings might show up in a BIG way and they might show up in a small way? Feelings might also show up in a way that feels nice or they might show up in a way that feels not so nice. For example, you might feel a "nice" nervous feeling right before your birthday party. Or you might feel "not so nice" nervous right before getting a flu shot at the doctor. What are the different ways you have felt nervous?

Materials:

- Journal or paper
- Drawing tools (crayons, colored pencils and/or markers)

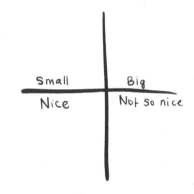

Steps:

1. Start by drawing a cross in your journal, so the page is divided into four sections.
2. "Nervous" is a very common feeling that we all can relate to, so let's start there. Use a section to draw a time when you felt big nervous, another to draw when you felt small nervous, and then "nice" and "not so nice nervous." Remind yourself that all feelings are ok and part of life!
3. If you have time, pick another emotion and explore this the same way.

Big picture questions:

1. Have you ever felt big nervous in a nice way? For example, if you learned you were going to Disneyland! How would that make you feel?
2. Have you felt small nervous in a nice way? How could you tell?
3. Sometimes it's hard to tell the difference between a nice feeling and a not so nice feeling. Why do you think that is?

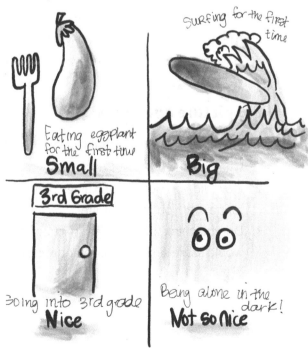

Student example

MEET A MARTIAN

Let's pretend that a spaceship landed on earth and a friendly Martian came out. He wants to know all about your life... What would you say? We have so many different things that make us unique. It's helpful to make art about what makes you, you! It can help us find people who share similar interests and it can also help us develop self-awareness to know who we are and what matters to us.

Materials:

- Journal or paper
- Drawing tools (crayons, colored pencils and/or markers)

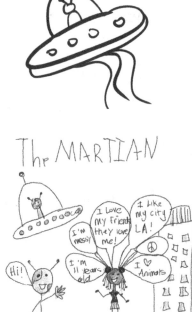

Steps:

1. First, set up the scene. What does the spaceship look like? Where has it landed? What do you think a Martian would look like? Be sure to draw yourself too.
2. Below your drawing, write what you would say to the Martian. Imagine yourself really there.
3. Here are some suggestions: My favorite color is... I like to... My favorite food is... Tell the Martian about your life. Where do you live? Who are your friends? What is the city the Martian landed in? Have fun, there's no wrong way to do it!

Student example

Big picture questions:

1. Of all the things you could say to the Martian, what would you most like to say?
2. How did you decide the things that are important about you and your life?
3. Do you think kids in other parts of the world would share similar or different things?

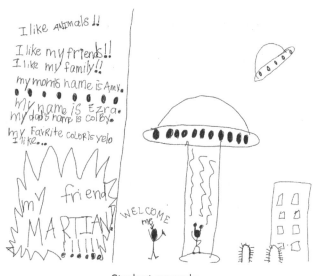

Student example

LIKES AND DISLIKES

You love chocolate but your best friend doesn't. You like sports but your brother prefers ballet. We all have different ways of seeing and experiencing things. It's curious the way we don't always agree. It can be fun and build self-awareness to reflect on your likes and dislikes. Let's practice this together with art.

Materials:

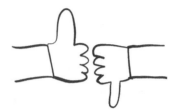

- Journal or paper
- Drawing tools (crayons, colored pencils and/or markers)

Steps:

1. Take a piece of paper and fold it in half.
2. On one side of the page, we will explore all of the things we like.
3. On the other side ... you guessed it, we will explore all the things we dislike.
4. As an exercise with your class, see if anyone drew the same thing as you.

Big picture questions:

1. Looking around the room, are there any similarities that you can see in our drawings today?
2. Do you think our likes and dislikes change as we get older? Why?
3. Have you ever thought you didn't like something, but then you tried it and everything changed?
4. Have you ever liked something, and then suddenly found you didn't like it anymore?
5. Do you notice if one side is easier than the other?

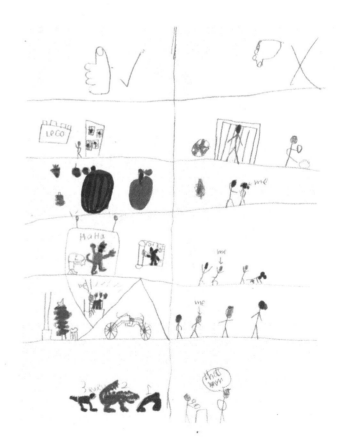

Student example

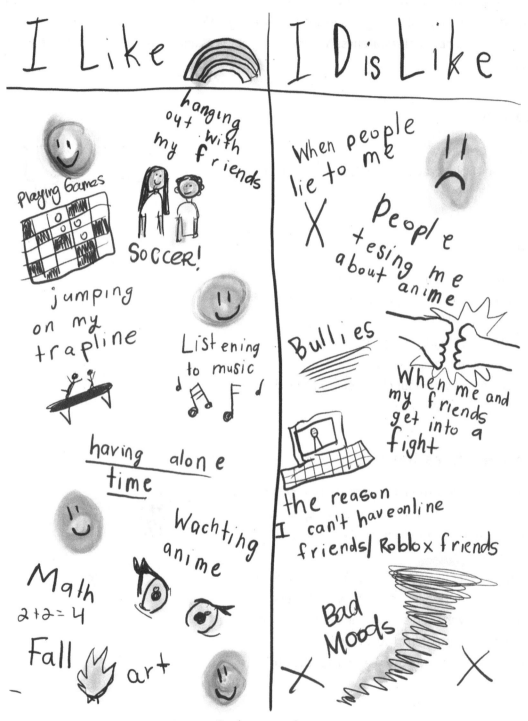

Student example

MY UNIQUE FAMILY

Every one of us is unique, with special experiences that make us who we are. We can learn a lot about ourselves from the people closest to us—like our family. In this exercise you will think of one special thing that you like about your family. For example, "My family and I love to go outside together and that's why I love nature!"

Materials:

- Journal or paper
- Drawing tools (crayons, colored pencils and/or markers)
- Scissors and glue

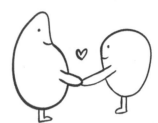

Steps:

1. Start by thinking about all the members of your family unit. Remember families come in all shapes and sizes. Friends can become part of our family too.
2. Cut out a shape, symbol or drawing to represent each person. There is no wrong way to do it! Is your aunt a square and your brother a triangle? Are you a star?
3. Think about the strengths your family has. For example, my family likes to laugh or my family plays sports together. Organize your shapes onto the page in any way you like and glue them down.

Big picture questions:

1. What symbols and shapes did you choose for your family? What made you choose them?
2. What is the symbol you chose for yourself in your family? Why?
3. Is there anything else to share about how you arranged the shapes and symbols of your family on the page?

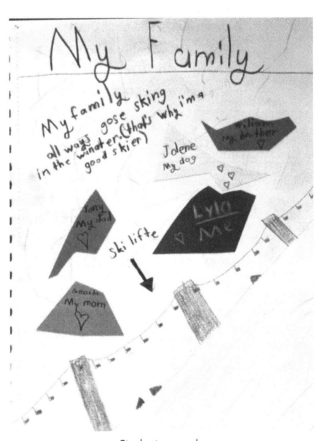

Student example

"TA-DA" LIST

You have heard of a "To-do" list, right? That's a list where you write down all of the things you want to accomplish. Well, a "ta-da" list is all about the things you have *already* done! It's important to remind ourselves of all the hard work we have put in and all the great things we have accomplished today.

Materials:

- Journal or paper
- Drawing tools (crayons, colored pencils and/or markers)

Steps:

1. Take a moment to think about all that you have accomplished today. Sometimes it's helpful to think about the little things, for example "I helped grandma with feeding our pet," or "I encouraged my friend to try something new."
2. You can make a list of all of the great things you have done today, or you can draw pictures.
3. Take a moment to reflect on all that you accomplished. How does that make you feel?

Big picture questions:

1. Why do we feel so good when we get things done?
2. Is there anything on your list that surprised you?
3. It feels nice to help others; does anyone have an example of how you helped a friend?

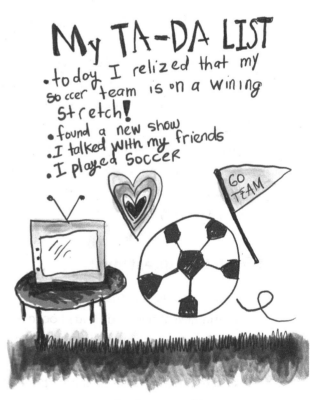

Student example

Chapter 2

SELF-MANAGEMENT

"I experimented with different brush strokes in my painting and found that I liked the feeling of moving the brush in different directions."

MIDDLE SCHOOL STUDENT

"My art is about peace. Anything within nature reminds me of my quiet place when I'm scared or sad. Nature makes me feel happy and I was inspired by the many colors found in nature. When I was little my dad and I would go out and catch butterflies and then let them go. It was relaxing to see them flap their wings and fly away..."

MIDDLE SCHOOL STUDENT

These two quotes, taken from a middle school art camp that we facilitated, illustrate how art can feel physically and emotionally calming. Manipulating different art materials like paint or clay can have a very peaceful effect even if you are not trying to make anything special. Using materials to represent different ideas can also shift a person's perspective to a place of relaxation.

Self-management is an important skill that helps people to manage thoughts, feelings and behaviors so that we can make good personal choices for ourselves in different types of situations. Self-management might look like impulse control, frustration tolerance, delaying gratification or managing stress in a healthy way. Self-management builds on self-awareness—now that students have figured out *how* they feel, self-management is about what they can *do* with those feelings.

I'm sure you're already thinking of many reasons why this SEL skill is so important! Practicing self-management can help kids to focus, resolve conflict in prosocial ways, persevere and reach personal goals. Self-management also includes increasing your ability to emotionally regulate. As we mentioned earlier, we like to think of emotional regulation or self-regulation like a thermostat; it's a tool for responding to the ups and downs of emotions.

Creating art independently or as a group is a great way to practice self-management!

As the two quotes shared above show, art-making is a great way to practice emotional regulation. Art materials can provide a sensory experience that can be calming to the body. Creating, or even just viewing, art can shift your students' perspectives and help them to think of things that could be more calming or pleasant.

In our work as art therapists, we learn that creating art in structures can offer containment and can provide students with opportunities to experience self-management and emotional regulation. For example, a third-grade teacher we worked with shared that the students were quite difficult to manage right after lunch. The teacher shared that he observed the students to be quite dysregulated, most likely due to the anxiety of returning to in-person situations after the pandemic and being isolated for so long. We suggested that the teacher offer his students materials such as stencils and gel pens, since these materials invite students to create in a structured boundary. The teacher reported back that the materials worked like magic to calm the students and help them focus on the next topic.

RAINBOW BREATHING

Let's practice building self-management by regulating with Rainbows! Taking deep breaths really helps our bodies to regulate—or find a sense of calm—so that we can make the best choices for ourselves. Can you think of a time when you were able to calm yourself? What did you do?

Materials:

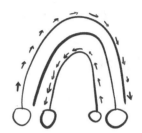

- Journal or paper
- Drawing tools (crayons, colored pencils and/or markers)

Steps:

1. Use your drawing tools to make a rainbow with big arches that fill your paper.
2. Once you have created your rainbow, use your finger to trace each line of the rainbow.
3. Breathe in as you go up and breathe out as you go down.
4. See what it feels like to go fast vs. slow.

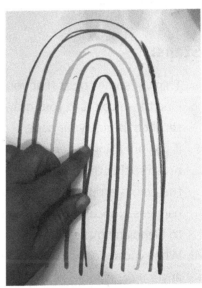

Big picture questions:

1. Practice breathing using your finger on the rainbow and without. What is the difference?
2. Do you think breathing is helpful when we are upset? Why?
3. When do you think it could be helpful to use your rainbow breathing art?

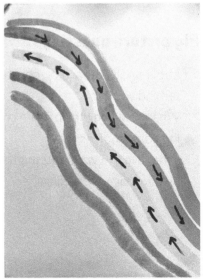

Student example

SOOTHING COLORS

What colors are soothing to you? Some people find the color blue soothing because it reminds them of water. Some people might choose the colors of the sunset. Someone else might like the colors we see in a forest. If everyone in the classroom made a painting of soothing colors, we might see a lot of the same, but also some very different interpretations. Making art with colors that you find soothing may help you feel a little bit calmer. Let's test it out!

Materials:

- Journal or paper
- Loose medium such as watercolor or paint
  (If paint is not an option, gluing down tissue paper works great too)

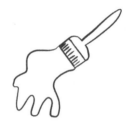

Steps:

1. Think of some colors that you find soothing.
2. Find those colors in your drawing materials and set them beside your paper.
3. If you are using watercolor, wet your pallet and brush so that the paint glides on the paper. Push the colors around on the paper and see what happens. Notice the parts where the paint begins to blend and make new colors.
4. When you are done, look around the room. Does anybody's art look like yours?

Big picture questions:

1. Looking at your color choices, what do they remind you of?
2. What would be the opposite color of your soothing color choice? Why?
3. What are the ways you might use this color to help manage big feelings?

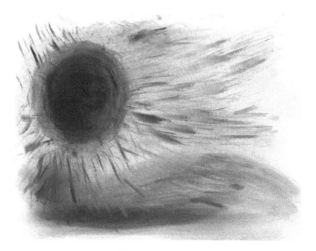

Student example

TORN PAPER COLLAGE

Our emotions and feelings can be all over the place. Lots of ups and lots of downs. Art is such a great way to help us regulate and keep our cool. For this exercise, let's try an art technique that can sometimes help relieve stress. Tearing paper using only your hands can help when you are feeling frustrated or angry. Being able to express your frustration in ways that are safe for you and others is an important life skill.

Materials:

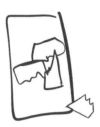

- Journal or paper
- A small collection of paper in different colors
- Repurposed paper like magazines, flyers and/or pamphlets
- Glue

Steps:

1. The steps for this activity are super easy. First, collect all of the colored paper and repurposed paper you have and select colors you find pleasing.
2. Rip your paper into strips and shapes.
3. Notice how it feels to not use scissors.
4. Keep going even if you get frustrated.
5. Have fun gluing your shapes down into any pleasing patterns you want.

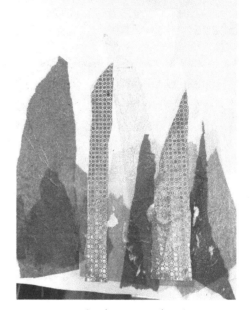

Student example

Big picture questions:

1. Describe how it feels to tear and rip the paper.
2. What are other ways that have helped you manage frustration?
3. How about when a friend or family member is frustrated? What can you do?

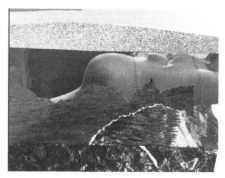

Student example

BEAUTIFUL BUBBLES!

What do a lot of people do right away when they see bubbles? POP them! It's almost as if they can't help it! Self-discipline is a skill that we practice to help us pause so that we can manage our bodies in healthy ways. For example, what if someone grabs a toy and we feel like hitting them? Or what would happen if we didn't pause and we ate a whole chocolate cake? Let's practice self-discipline by creating a beautiful bubble maze where we practice going around bubbles instead of popping them!

Materials:

- Journal or paper
- Crayons, colored pencils, markers
- (Optional: watercolor paint palette, brushes, water)

Steps:

1. In your journal or on a piece of paper using drawing tools or watercolor paint, fill your page with beautiful bubbles!
2. After you have created your bubbles, use drawing tools or watercolor paint to make marks or fill in the areas around the bubbles—careful!
3. Use self-discipline to go slowly so you don't "pop" the bubble!
4. If you have time, you and a partner can make another bubble maze, or switch and practice self-discipline by going around each other's bubbles!

Big picture questions:

1. What is an example of a time you practiced self-discipline?
2. What thoughts or actions did you use to help you?
3. Why do you think self-discipline might be important? For kids? For adults?

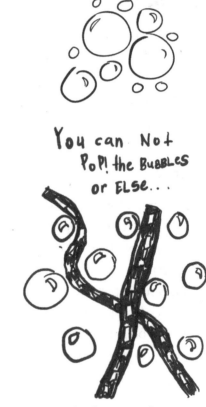

Student example

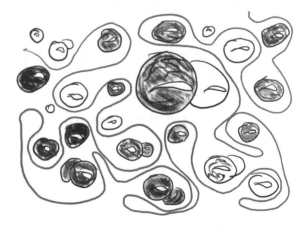

Student example

LIBRARY OF CALM

Being aware of what we find calming is an important tool that helps us to calm our bodies, regulate our emotions and make good choices for ourselves. A library is a place where information is kept for people to use. Let's do some research and create our own library of what we find calming for each of our five senses!

Materials:

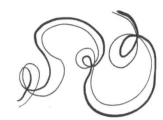

- Journal or paper
- Drawing tools (crayons, colored pencils and/or markers)

Steps:

1. Create a table in your journal that has six spaces; one for your name and the other five for your senses: sight, sound, taste, touch, smell.
2. Close your eyes or find somewhere to gaze and take three big deep breaths.
3. Think back to a time or times when you felt very calm and relaxed. What do you remember? What do you remember seeing? What did it sound like? What are the tastes and smells that you remember? What were you touching?
4. Use drawing tools to draw things that you find calming to each of your five senses.

Big picture questions:

1. Can you think of a time or place when *all five* of your senses were calm? Describe it in as much detail as you can.
2. Sometimes just *thinking* about things that are calming can help your body relax. When might this be a helpful tool?

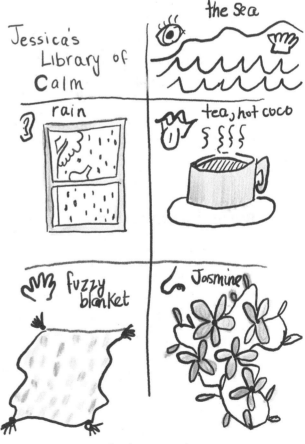

Student example

AFFIRMATION STATION

Affirmations are things that we can say to ourselves when we feel challenged by a thought, feeling or situation. Affirmations are positive, encouraging and personally meaningful words or phrases like "I can do this" or "I am loved." They can be important tools in helping us to manage our thoughts and feelings in ways that feel good and help us overcome challenges. Can you think of an affirmation you can use?

Materials:

- Journal or paper
- Colored pencils or crayons
- Watercolor paint palette, brushes, water
- (Optional: watercolor paper)

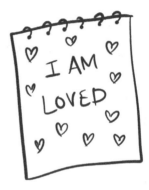

Steps:

1. Take a moment to think about a time when you felt challenged. What do you remember thinking or feeling? What did you think or say to yourself that helped you keep going? ·
2. Discuss with a friend or share with the class.
3. Write the words or draw a symbol that represents your affirmation.
4. Decorate your affirmation with lines, shapes, colors or paint over the words or symbols with watercolor paint.

Big picture questions:

1. Affirmations are a popular way to provide support. What are other affirmations that you've heard at school, in movies or at events?
2. Share your affirmation with a partner. Have them say it to you. How does it feel? Now switch.

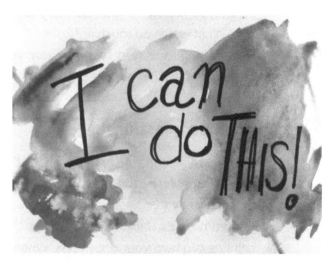

Student example

THE POWER OF YET!

Having a "growth mindset" means that you focus not on what you can't do but on what you CAN do with practice and hard work. When we are struggling to learn a new skill, changing our words can help us to keep going. Instead of saying, "I can't ride a bike," try, "I can't ride a bike YET." What are you learning right now? What are some of the steps that you can take on your "YET" journey?

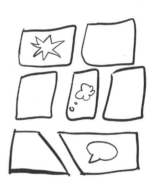

Materials:

- Journal or paper
- Drawing tools (crayons, colored pencils and/or markers)

Steps:

1. Think of something that you are learning right now but maybe feel challenged by, for example, roller skating, reading, swimming?
2. Try changing your language to include "yet," i.e. "I can't roller skate YET."
3. What are some of the steps you could take on your journey of YET?
4. In your journal or on a piece of paper divide the page into sections—like a comic strip!
5. In the first box, draw yourself trying the skill you're learning.
6. In the last box, draw yourself accomplishing the skill. In the boxes in between, draw some of the steps you can take on your "yet" journey.
7. Take a moment to share with the class, how does that make you feel?

Big picture questions:

1. Think about the "Affirmation Station" activity. What are some affirmations that might help you on your journey of YET?
2. Sometimes it's helpful to have someone to practice a new skill with. Who is someone you might include on your journey of YET?
3. Is there a way that you could motivate yourself on your journey? A special prize or treat?

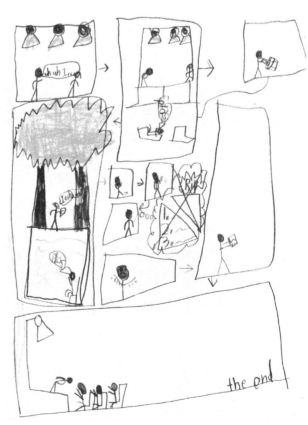

Student example

49

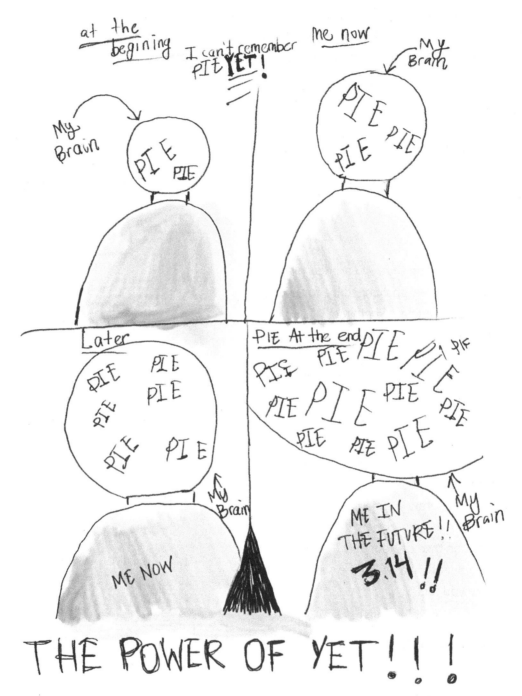

Student example

COOL AS A CUCUMBER!

Have you ever heard the phrase "cool as a cucumber"? Being "cool as a cucumber" is a silly phrase that means being calm and regulated. Sometimes repeating a calming phrase or picturing a calming or silly image can help us when we are finding it difficult to manage tough feelings. Let's create our own "cool cucumber" that we can think of when we're feeling not so calm.

Materials:

- Journal or paper
- Drawing tools (crayons, colored pencils and/or markers)

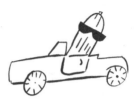

Steps:

1. Think of what makes you feel cool and calm.
2. How would this feeling look as a cucumber? Would the cucumber be wearing sunglasses? Sipping a cool lemonade? Maybe floating in a refreshing pool?
3. Be silly and let your imagination go to create your own cool cucumber.
4. If comfortable, share your image with a classmate. Hang the cucumbers up in your classroom to remind one another that there are lots of ways to be a "cool cucumber"!

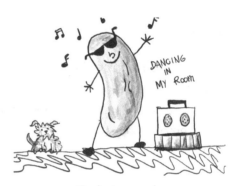

Student example

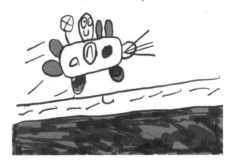

Student example

Big picture questions:

1. Take a look at some of your peers' "cool cucumbers." What are some of the similarities?
2. Can you think of anyone in your life or in the movies that reminds you of a "cool cucumber"? How do you think they keep their "cool"?
3. Has there ever been a time that you were acting like a "cool cucumber" but inside you were feeling really nervous? Did acting like a "cool cucumber" help? Is it a useful strategy for you to use in nervous moments?

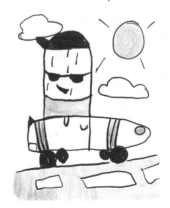

Student example

RELAXING WITH MUSIC

Music is a wonderful way to regulate our emotions when we're feeling challenged by a thought, feeling or situation. Combining art-making and music creates even more opportunities to relax and regulate. What type of music do you find relaxing?

Materials:

■ Journal or paper
■ Colored pencils or crayons
■ Watercolor paint palette, brushes, water
■ (Optional: watercolor paper)

Steps:

1. Collect your choice of art-making tools (colored pencils, crayons or watercolor).
2. Find an empty page in your journal or a piece of watercolor paper.
3. Take a deep breath, close your eyes or gaze lightly.
4. Play music. Listen for a few moments. How do you feel? If the music were a color what would it be? What type of line? Shape?
5. Begin drawing or painting what the music looks like to you using lines, shapes and/or colors.

Big picture questions:

1. Take a look at your image. What do you see? How does it make you feel?
2. Take a look at your image again. How would you move around the image? Where would you start? Where would you end?
3. What type of movements might match your image?

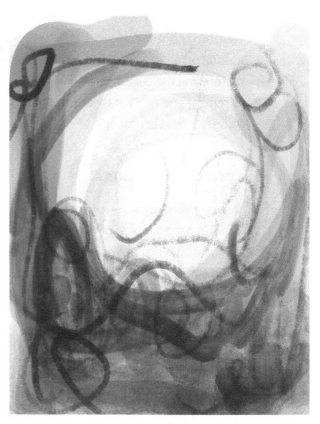

Student example

EMOTIONAL ENVIRONMENT

When we have big emotions, it can feel like we are surrounded by them or stuck in them! Sometimes it's hard to see our way out. Thinking about what the feeling or emotion might look like might help give us clues for how to manage the emotion and get unstuck! Can you imagine one of your emotions as an environment or landscape? What might help you in this environment?

Materials:

- Journal or paper
- Colored pencils or crayons
- Watercolor paint palette, brushes, water
- (Optional: watercolor paper, colored paper, glue)

Steps:

1. Think of an emotion or feeling that has challenged you. Anger? Sadness? Fear?
2. If it were an environment, what would it look like? The bottom of a volcano? Maybe being caught in a thunderstorm?
3. Use drawing, painting or torn paper to create this environment.
4. Take a step back and look at your image.
5. What tools might a person need in this environment? A fireproof suit? An umbrella? Use your drawing tools to add these tools to the environment.
6. Share with the class or a person sitting nearby. Do they have ideas for what a person would need in this environment?

Big picture questions:

1. Taking a look at your image, think about where you might be in the landscape or environment? Describe how it feels. Describe how it feels to use the tools you included.
2. Imagine yourself moving to a different environment or landscape. What would it look like?

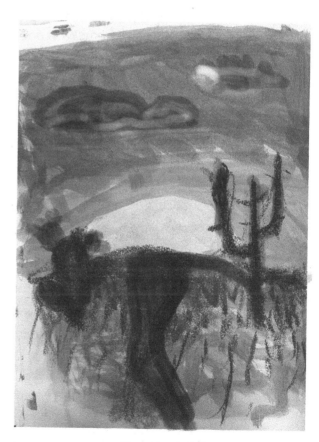

Student example

CREATURE TEACHER

Getting to know our feelings is an important skill that can help us learn what we need when we are having a feeling, for example, feeling sad and needing a hug or feeling frustrated and needing some space. Exploring our feelings in a funny way can help us practice sitting with and managing our feelings. What would one of your feelings look like if it was a creature? What can this creature help you learn about yourself?

Materials:

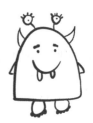

- Journal or paper
- Colored pencils or crayons

Steps:

1. Think about a feeling that you want to get to know a little better: anger, sadness, fear, frustration, silliness.
2. Think about some characteristics this feeling might have. What does it wear or eat? Where does it live? Where is it from? What does it like to do? Who are its friends? What does it sound like?
3. Use your imagination and draw what your feeling would look like if it were a creature.
4. Think about what this creature might need.
5. Use drawing tools to create an environment for your creature.
6. Share your creature with your class or someone sitting close by. Ask questions about other people's creatures.

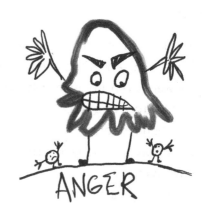

Student example

Big picture questions:

1. What did you learn about the feeling you chose?
2. How does your creature make you think differently about the feeling you chose?

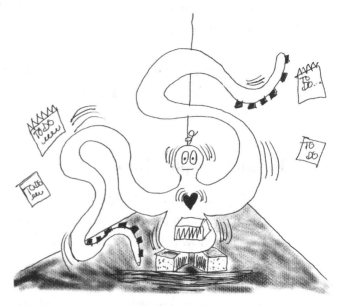

Student example

WARM AND COOL COLORS

We can use Warm and Cool Colors in our art to explore and express our moods and feelings. Finding different ways to express ourselves can help us manage our feelings in a positive way. For this activity we will make a landscape drawing using only warm colors on one side—that's red, orange and yellow. On the other side, you will color the image using only cool colors—that's purple, blue and green.

Materials:

- Journal or paper
- Colored pencils or crayons
- (Optional: watercolor paint palette, brushes, water)

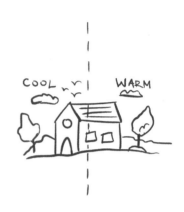

Steps:

1. Decide on a landscape that you would like to choose for your drawing. A landscape is a picture of something outside, like the ocean, or a mountain scene, a cityscape, the desert, or a cabin in the forest.
2. Fold your paper in half so there is a line down the middle.
3. On one side you will add color to your drawing with only warm colors and on the other side you will use only cool colors.

Big picture questions:

1. Think about the process of making your image. What was easy? What was challenging?
2. Take a moment to look at your image. What type of emotions and/or feelings might be represented on each side? Is there a story that goes with it?

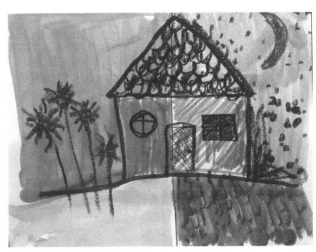

Student example

Chapter 3

SOCIAL AWARENESS

"Creating art with my child allowed me to communicate in ways that I haven't yet before. Through art we were able to open up about how we felt and that had very deep meaning. We were able to have in depth conversations after our sessions from our artwork and, overall, it brought us closer."

ART WORKSHOP PARENT ATTENDEE

Whereas self-awareness is about getting to know yourself, social awareness is about developing an awareness of others. Social awareness is a skill that is about developing empathy and compassion for others by considering different perspectives. Social awareness might look like the ability to recognize feelings in others, consider someone else's point of view, show concern for others and appreciate unique differences.

The skill of social awareness is not just important for the individual but also for our communities as a whole! Creating spaces for children to cultivate their natural tendencies towards empathy can help them to manage conflict more effectively as well as be more sensitive and open to cultural differences.

Creating and sharing art provides so many fantastic ways for students to practice social awareness! Creating art offers opportunities to witness and learn about why classmates created what they did. Asking questions and engaging in dialogue about why each student made the artistic choices they made can create an increased awareness about self and others.

The way that we talk and ask questions about artwork is a fantastic opportunity to build social awareness. Continuing to practice curiosity about why we made what we made increases our self-awareness *and* our social awareness. Remember to do your best to encourage your students to refrain from making value-based statements about an artist's work but to instead show curiosity and ask questions. Here are a couple of starter questions and comments we've found to really elicit some reflection and connection amongst young artists:

- "I see..."
- "I wonder...?"
- "Can you tell me more about...?"
- "Is there a story about ...?"

BILLBOARD ABOUT ME

Being aware and confident in who you are as well as what you value and believe is an important social skill to practice. Letting people know what's important about you—and just as important, to also listen to the things that are important to them—will help you build healthy relationships. A billboard is a large sign that shares information for many people to see. Let's create a billboard about you! What is important to know about you?

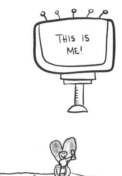

Materials:

- Journal or paper
- Drawing tools (crayons, colored pencils and/or markers)
- (Optional: a rectangle to trace)

Steps:

1. Start by brainstorming all the things that are important to you.
2. Write them in your journal or talk as a class or with a friend.
3. Once you have identified things that are important to you, draw or trace a rectangle in the middle of your page
4. Create a billboard that shares important information about you!
5. When finished, take turns sharing your billboards with a friend or as a class. Remember to listen when others are sharing.

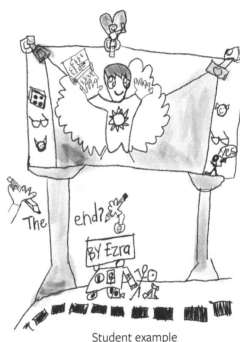

Student example

Big picture questions:

1. When you look around the room, do you see any similarities?
2. Let's take a moment to get curious about what we see on the billboard of our friends. Is anyone curious about something they see here?
3. One key aspect of social awareness is taking on the perspective of another person. Do you think we came to a better understanding about each other? Why?

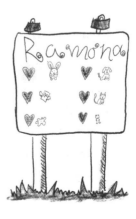

Student example

WHAT STORIES WILL YOU TELL?

When we organize and plan carefully, we can accomplish great things. Let's put this into action by following the steps to fold a mini book. This activity takes patience and sometimes you might find that you need to start over. Once you get it right, you will be able to make lots of tiny books to tell all your stories!

Materials:

- Loose paper (printer paper works great)
- Any mark-making tools you would like to work with
- Scissors
- Glue stick
- Paper scraps (e.g. magazines)

Steps:

1. Get yourself ready to watch the teacher very closely as they show you the steps to fold your mini book.
2. Listen carefully and follow the instructions.
3. If you don't get it right the first time, keep trying and stay patient. It can take some practice sometimes.
4. Use colored construction paper, markers and/or colored pencils to create images on the pages of your book.
5. What stories will you tell? Perhaps you can make a lot of stories to share with your friends.

Big picture questions:

1. Would anyone like to share their story today?
2. Storytelling is a long-standing tradition in many, many cultures. Why do you think people like to share stories with each other?
3. Does your story say anything about you and what is important to you? Why?

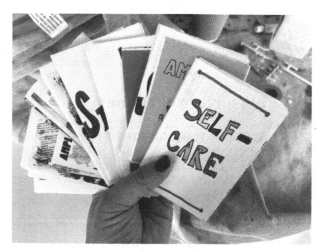

Student example

WHO ARE YOUR HELPERS?

Knowing who we can trust and who in our community makes us feel safe is an important skill. We can call these people helpers. Who are helpers in your community? How many helpers can you think of?

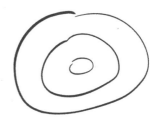

Materials:

- Journal or paper
- Drawing tools (crayons, colored pencils and/or markers)
- (Optional: circular objects to trace)

Steps:

1. Draw or trace a small circle in the middle of your page and write your name and/or draw a symbol that represents you in the center.
2. Draw or trace a second circle around this circle and write the names and/or draw symbols for all the helpers you have in your community: your family, pets, teachers, doctors, mail carriers, garbage collectors—the list can go on and on!
3. Draw or trace one more circle around the outside circle. In this circle, write or draw how you are a helper.
4. When you are finished, share with a neighbor or as a class. Are there other helpers you can add?

Big picture questions:

1. Why do we need helpers in our communities?
2. How do you express gratitude to the helpers around you?
3. Can you think of the last time you helped someone? What happened? How did they feel? How did you feel?

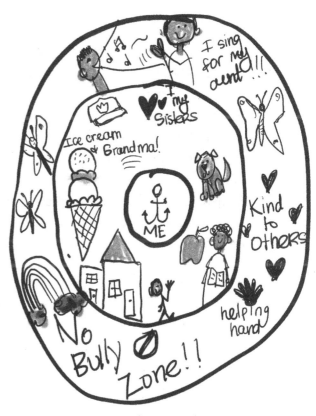

Student example

SETTING THE STAGE FOR RESILIENCE

The word resilient means being able to bounce back and get through hard stuff. Can you think of a time when you felt challenged? Maybe it was really uncomfortable or scary, but you got through it! Sometimes, we have to build ourselves up to set the stage for resilience. It's like bringing forward a super brave part of ourselves. Pretending you're brave can actually help you to feel brave. Let's have fun imagining you were a brave character in a play. What does your brave, resilient self look like?

Materials:

- Journal or paper
- Drawing tools (crayons, colored pencils and/or markers)

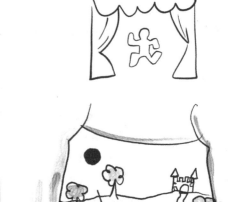

Steps:

1. Imagine a time you felt really brave. Or you can remember a time when you saw someone else being really brave, either in real life or a movie. What did this person look like? If you were playing the role of a brave person in a play or movie, what kind of costume would you pick?
2. Do your best to draw a stage and add yourself to it complete with a brave, resilient costume!
3. Big picture questions:
4. As we look at the images our friends have made around the room, we can see many strengths. Can you let someone know what you see in their drawing that represents a strength.
5. Sometimes when we have an obstacle in front of us, we have an opportunity to grow. Can you think of an example?

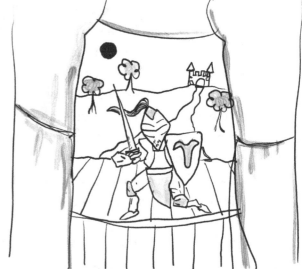

Student example

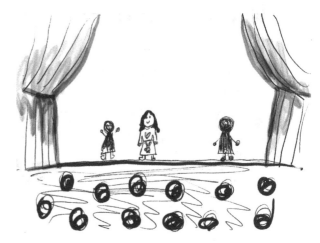

Student example

A MILE IN YOUR SHOES

Being able to understand someone else's perspective is an important skill that will help you develop great relationships and have empathy—a skill that helps you think about another person's feelings or experiences. The phrase "to really know someone is to walk a mile in their shoes" describes how we can put ourselves in someone else's position to understand their experience. Let's work with a classmate to see what a mile in their shoes might look like!

Materials:

- Journal or paper
- Drawing tools (crayons, colored pencils and/or markers)

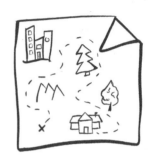

Steps:

1. Find a partner and interview them about their day.
2. Where do they begin their day, what do they do in the middle of their day and where do they end their day? Be sure to really listen to all the details.
3. Using drawing tools create a map that shows how your partner spends their day.
4. Draw their home, how they might get to school, what they do after school and where they might go to end their day.
5. Make sure to share with your partner and check-in to see if you understood them correctly.
6. Switch so that you each get a turn drawing. Have fun!

Big picture questions:

1. What is something new you learned about your partner?
2. How did you feel when you shared your day with your partner?
3. What were the similarities and differences in your day?

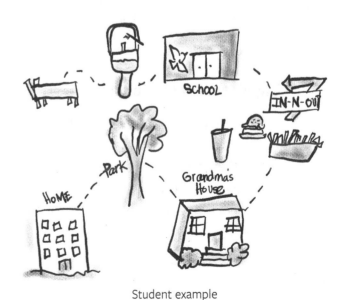

Student example

ROLE MODEL COLLAGE

When you think about a person you really respect, you are identifying qualities that you aspire to. Exploring the impact others have on people will help you connect with how you might impact others around you. Our activity today invites you to think about someone you look up to. It can be anyone: your soccer coach, your uncle, your friend's older sister. Maybe there is a fellow student in your classroom.

Materials:

- Journal or paper
- Magazine scraps
- Scissors
- Glue

Steps:

1. Flip through the magazine images and pick an image that reminds you of your role model. It doesn't have to look at all like them but rather have some quality that makes you think of them.
2. Cut out the image, arrange it and glue it on a piece of paper.
3. Add some color and words too to represent the qualities you admire in this person.
4. Share with the person next to you why you look up to this person.

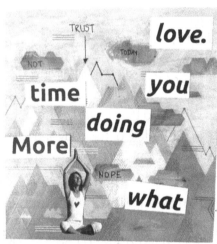

Student example

Big picture questions:

1. Who did you choose to represent on your page? Why?
2. Are there any qualities about them that you see in yourself? Why?
3. In what ways would you like to be like them?

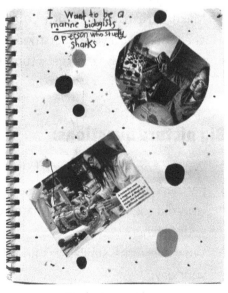

Student example

COMING TO THE TABLE

Understanding that everyone has different experiences that affect the way they think, feel and act is important in building social awareness. Food and certain meals can have a lot of significance or importance to a person. Meals can include important memories or traditions that we cherish. Many cultures come together to share a meal on special occasions like birthdays, holidays or weddings. What is a meal that you can think of that helps you come together with others?

Materials:

- Journal or paper, colored construction paper
- Drawing tools (crayons, colored pencils and/or markers)
- (Optional: magazine collage images, scissors and glue sticks)

Steps:

1. Think of, list or discuss foods and/or meals that are important to your family. Why are these foods or meals important? Who makes this meal? How and who do you share this meal with?
2. In your journal or on a piece of paper, do your best to draw a plate.
3. Use your drawing tools or magazine collage images to create a meal that is important to your family.
4. Bring your image to the carpet or a large table where you can share your family meal with the class. Remember to really listen to what others share!

Big picture questions:

1. Food has a lot to do with where we come from and who we are. In what ways does your meal represent you?
2. Many of our favorite foods are tied to traditions. When do you eat your special meal?
3. Is there anything else you would like to share about your meal?

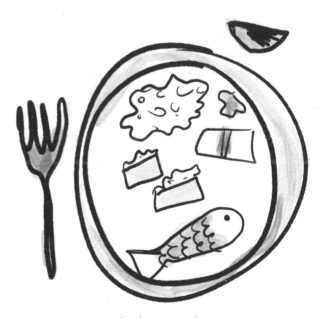

Student example

RECIPE FOR A GREAT DAY

If you were going to have the best day ever what would that look like? Thinking about what we need to help us feel good is a great skill for social awareness! If we are aware of the things we need to have a great day we are more likely to make those things happen! Some examples could be getting enough sleep, eating a good breakfast or spending time with friends that help you feel good. What are all the ingredients you need to have a great day?

Materials:

- Journal or paper
- Drawing tools (crayons, colored pencils and/or markers)

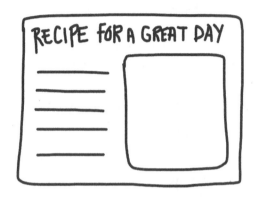

Steps:

1. Think about the last time you had a great day and/or think about what would make a great day for you.
2. List all the things or ingredients you need to make that day great.
3. Draw a picture that shows this great day.

Big picture questions:

1. What are the things you need for your great day?
2. Do you see any similarities with some of your friends here?
3. What are some other recipes we can think of? A recipe for our classroom? Or how about a recipe for feeling calm, or a recipe for feeling happy? Let's work together to create more recipes.

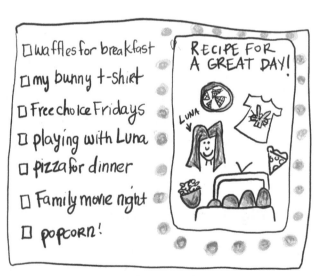

Student example

A HELPING HAND

Showing concern for others is an important skill that benefits everyone. When we show support and feel support from our community it can help us feel safe and calm. We can show support in lots of different ways. We can use our words, our bodies, or our actions to show support. How do you show support?

Materials:

- Journal or paper
- Drawing tools (crayons, colored pencils and/or markers)

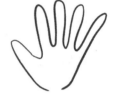

Steps:

1. In your journal or on a piece of paper, using a drawing tool, trace the outline of your hand.
2. Inside the outline of your hand, use images, symbols, lines, shapes or colors to represent all the ways that you show concern for a friend, classmate or community member.
3. If comfortable, share your work with a classmate. How does your classmate show concern? How do they like to receive concern?

Big picture questions:

1. Why does it feel good to help others?
2. How do you think it feels for others when they are helped by someone?
3. Would you like to share an idea of how you can help others more in the future?

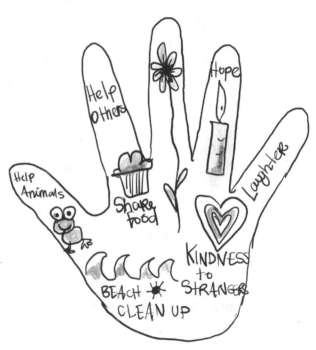

Student example

GRATITUDE GARLAND

Gratitude means being thankful! Giving thanks for the qualities we appreciate about ourselves and others is a great way to create a positive classroom environment. Let's think of all the things we appreciate about each other and create a garland to decorate your space!

Materials:

- Journal or paper
- Drawing tools (crayons, colored pencils and/or markers)
- String, yarn, long strip of paper
- Tape

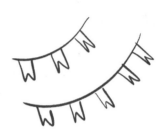

Steps:

1. Begin by thinking of, discussing or listing all the things you are thankful about yourself and your classmates or friends.
2. Using different shapes of paper and drawing tools, create images and words to show gratitude.
3. Attach all the shapes to a string, yarn or long strip of paper.
4. In your journal or on a piece of paper, do your best to draw a prize ribbon or a trophy shape.
5. Fill your shape with words, images, lines, shapes or color to represent your unique skills or talents.
6. If comfortable, share with a classmate or class, or hang awards in the classroom for all to share! Celebrate the similarities and the differences!

Big picture questions:

1. How will we all feel if we continue to have this "gratitude attitude" with each other?
2. What might be different and special about our class if we continue to share empathy and compassion with each other?

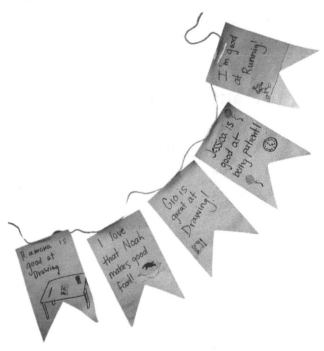

Student example

R-E-S-P-E-C-T (SELF AND OTHERS)

Respect. What does that word mean? Well, it means a lot of things and you probably hear grown-ups use it a lot. In a nutshell, respect means showing you care. That you care about how your words and actions affect others. That you care about how you treat yourself. That you can find ways to demonstrate kindness even when you disagree or feel frustrated by something. That you can find ways to show yourself compassion and kindness too.

Materials:

- Journal or paper
- Drawing tools (crayons, colored pencils and/or markers)

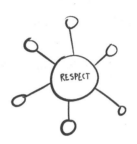

Steps:

1. Brainstorm with your class all the ways we can show others respect in our classroom by making a spider map like the one pictured above. See, it kind of looks like a spider!
2. Next draw pictures or examples about how that might look in your classroom.
3. You can make your own spider map, or you and your class can make a huge spider map for your classroom wall so you can all remember how to demonstrate respect at school.
4. If you finish your spider map, draw a picture of all the people in your classroom.

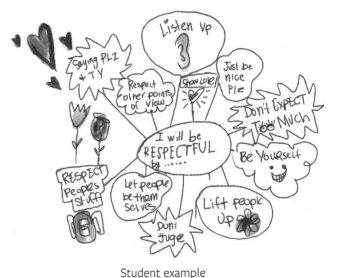

Student example

Big picture questions:

1. What are some of the ideas that you chose to represent on your page?
2. How can we help our classroom show up for others with respect?

CELEBRATING OUR VALUES!

Things can be hard sometimes. But even when we have difficult things we must go through, we can always think of people in our lives who encourage us to remember our values and the things that are important to us. Let's celebrate the people in our lives who encourage us to be the best we can be.

Materials:

- Journal or paper
- Drawing tools (crayons, colored pencils and/or markers)
- (Optional: colored paper, scissors and glue)

Steps:

1. Draw large confetti pieces filling up your page for your celebration.
2. In the confetti shapes, write down some of the names of people in your life who encourage you to remember what you value. Write down some of your values too. For example, love, kindness, compassion, friendship etc.
3. Have fun filling up your page with fun colors. You can use colorful paper and scissors to make more confetti.

Big picture questions:

1. Who are you celebrating with your confetti pieces?
2. Do we see any similarities?
3. Share why you chose your people if you like.

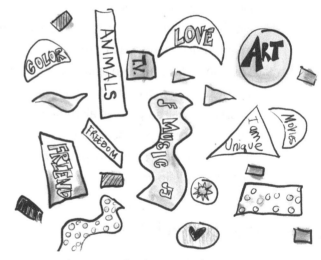

Student example

Chapter 4

RELATIONSHIP SKILLS

"I didn't like talking, I didn't like being a part of anything, everyone remembers me as the girl with my hair over my face. [By participating in the summer workshop] I realized it was the way I was able to express myself that was helping me form strong bonds and realize that my words meant a lot. It all had a great impact on how I am today."

STUDENT PARTICIPANT OF ART WORKSHOP REFLECTING ON HER EXPERIENCE YEARS LATER

This quote is from a former student attendee reflecting back 15 years after her first experience making art during a summer arts workshop. She states that it was exploring her creativity in the group setting that helped her open up to making new friends. This is a perfect model of how relationship skills can be enhanced through collaborative art-making and can encourage students to feel seen and heard in group settings.

Relationship skills are important in developing lasting friendships, learning about self and others, asking for help when needed and building social support within our communities. When we attend to our relationships, we develop important communication skills that help us with conflict resolution and problem-solving.

Making your classroom a place where people feel safe and have good relationships can build a sense of trust which then enables people to be vulnerable with each other. It can unite your classroom through shared values which can lead to growth in other contexts like academics or school pride and engagement. Creating this sense of trust can influence positive risk-taking, which might look like opening up about a shared struggle, raising a hand to share in discussion or being an upstander to unkind or unsafe behavior.

Bonding through the art process is organic and effortless. It's a great way to get students talking about their likes and dislikes and can offer a visual aid that helps students open up to others about their personal experiences. Alternatively, art doesn't always have to be serious. Art can also support bonding by creating opportunities to be silly and playful together. As we have illustrated in the previous chapters, art directives do not need to be focused on personal matters to get students to warm up, there are many low-risk art activities that can support cooperation and teamwork.

Consider using your recipes to partner up students. This will be a chance to support cooperation and teamwork. If you establish smaller groups, when it is time to share about their process, you may create a safer space to share for the quieter voices in your classroom. It can be interesting to change things up in your groups. For example, intentionally leaving a material out like a pencil and a ruler could offer students an added challenge to plan things out before officially marking or gluing pieces down.

BUGGING OUT

What really "bugs" you in life? Thinking about the things that bug us can help us get more in touch with the things that irritate us and cause our emotional temperature to rise. When we do this, we can then know to avoid certain situations or that we will need to practice our skills to get through annoying situations that can't be avoided. For example, it might really bug you when your little brother takes forever to buckle his seatbelt, but you breathe through it because you know he's little. What really "bugs" you?

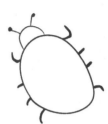

Materials:

- Journal or paper
- Drawing tools (crayons, colored pencils and/or markers)

Steps:

1. Draw a bug, any bug, as big as you can on the page.
2. Use the center of the space to explore some of the things that really annoy you. For example, when your little sister takes your stuff, waking up early in the morning or when Mom says no!
3. Share about your drawing with the person next to you. See if there are any similarities or differences.
4. Offering validation to others is a kind act to do for a classmate. That might look like nodding your head and saying you understand. It might sound like this: "I hear that _____ really bugs you, that must be very frustrating. Is there anything that helps you through it?"

Big picture questions:

1. Sometimes we find things really annoying and other times just a little? How do you decide which is which?
2. What are some of the strategies you use when you are feeling bugged?
3. How might it be helpful to learn about what your peers are bugged by?

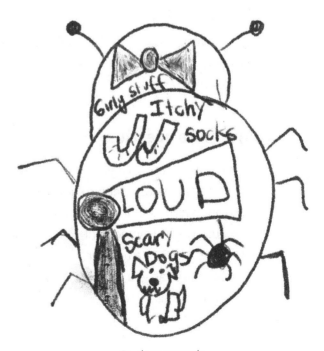

Student example

MY CULTURAL LENS

The word "culture" is a word that describes a big idea! Culture describes all the ways a person lives their life! This includes the food we eat, the things we celebrate, the clothes we wear or the languages we speak! Our culture shapes the way we see ourselves and interact in our world. Being aware of our unique culture and how it affects the way we see our world is very important. Let's explore how culture shapes what we see by creating a cultural lens!

Materials:

- Journal or paper
- Drawing tools (crayons, colored pencils and/or markers)
- (Optional: clear transparency and pastels)

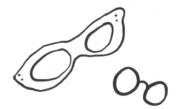

Steps:

1. Start by thinking about all the ways you live your life... What do you eat? Wear? What games/sports do you play? What things do you celebrate?
2. Try your best to draw a pair of glasses.
3. Draw images, symbols, lines, shapes or colors in the lenses to represent the many different pieces of your culture.
4. If comfortable, share with a classmate. What do you have in common? What is different? Imagine what it might be like to look through someone else's cultural lens?

Big picture questions:

1. Think about the things that are important to your culture. Would people know just by looking at you that these things were important?
2. Discuss why it is important to learn about culture? As a kid? As a teacher?
3. What things can you do to learn about your own or someone else's culture?

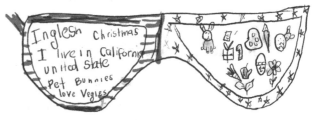

Student example

IF YOU KNEW US, YOU WOULD KNOW...

Identity is a word that is similar to the word culture that describes all the unique things that make you, you! Sometimes the most important things about our identity are things that are not seen by others right away. Let's take some time to think about some of the things that make up our unique identities—especially the things that people may not notice right away!

Materials:

- Journal or paper
- Drawing tools (crayons, colored pencils and/or markers)

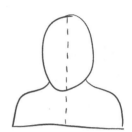

Steps:

1. Begin by quietly considering the prompt, "If you knew me you would know..." Write or think about all the unique things that make you, you. For example, "If you knew me you would know that my favorite color is green, I have two little sisters, a cat named Sox, and I only eat the tops off my broccoli."
2. Next, share responses you are comfortable sharing with a friend/classmate.
3. Work together on a piece of paper to do your best to draw a circle or the shape of a head and divide it in half.
4. Continue to work together to fill in one half each with words, images, lines, shapes and/or colors that represent both of you.
5. If comfortable, share with the class!

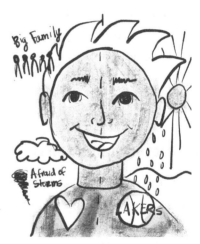

Student example

Big picture questions:

1. What did you learn about your partner? What were the similarities and/or differences?
2. Think about the process of creating your image with another person. What was the experience like?
3. Why do you think it might be helpful to learn about your identity? How could that help your relationships?

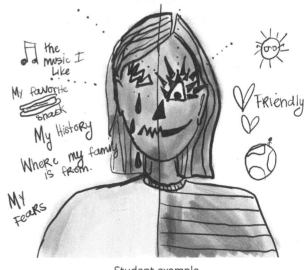

Student example

75

BEING A FRIEND

Sometimes the smallest of gestures can make us feel better when we're having a tough day. It's important to be there for others because it gives us a sense of purpose and helps us build strong and lasting friendships. Reflect on a time when someone was kind to you and how it made you feel better. How could you be a good friend?

Materials:

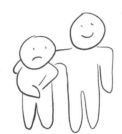

- Journal or paper
- Drawing tools (crayons, colored pencils and/or markers)

Steps:

1. Split your paper in half so we can think about two scenarios.
2. On one side of the page, draw a person having a bad day.
3. On the other side of the page, draw how you could be a good friend.

Big picture questions:

1. Look around at your classmates' images. What are some ways to be a good friend?
2. What are things that might make it hard to be a good friend? What can you do to make it easier?
3. Are there different things you might do for different friends? Share examples if you are comfortable.

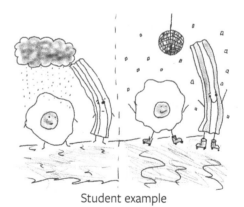

Student example

MAKE YOUR CHOICE

Conflict is when we disagree, argue or fight with another person. Conflict happens to everyone and is a natural part of relationships. If we stop and reflect, conflict can help us learn how we want to be treated and how to treat others. There are lots of choices for how to handle conflict in a positive way when it arises. Being aware of what choices work for you can help you grow in your relationships. What are some choices you can make when you have a relationship conflict?

Materials:

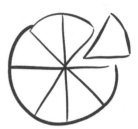

- Journal or paper
- Drawing tools (crayons, colored pencils and/or markers)
- (Optional: circular object to trace)

Steps:

1. Write in your journal or brainstorm as a class all the choices you have when relationship conflict happens, e.g. talk it out, use "I statements," walk away, apologize, ask for help, compromise.
2. Draw or trace a circle in your journal or on your paper and divide the circle into sections.
3. In each section write or draw symbols that represent all the different choices you can make when relationship conflict happens.

Big picture questions:

1. What choice do you often make when you have conflict?
2. What choices are harder? Easier?
3. How can a relationship grow as a result of conflict?

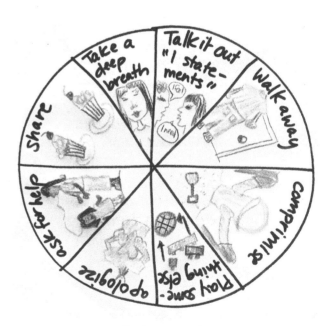

Student example

LEADERSHIP LIGHT

We all have a light that shines within us and one of the best ways for us to bring light into our community is to help others find their light. The light in me can help the light in "we." Let's think about your light and all that you have to offer others. For example, your great sense of humor helps others find laughter! When you find your light, you can lead by example.

Materials:

- Journal or paper
- Drawing tools (crayons, colored pencils and/or markers)

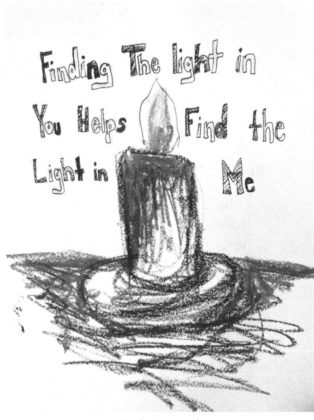

Steps:

1. Do your best to draw a lightbulb, a flashlight, a lantern, a candle, a lamp or any other tool that shines bright light so we can see when things get dark.
2. Brainstorm how you can lead others by using your strengths.
3. Spend some time drawing about how sharing your strengths with others can help shine light in the community.
4. When you are done, put all of your lights together. Just think about how bright this light will be!

Big picture questions:

1. What are some of the strengths you identified in your drawing?
2. How might your strengths be combined with others in your class?
3. Who are other people in your community that share their leadership light?

Student example

COLLABORATIVE DRAWING

When we work with others, we get to share our ideas. The word collaborate means to work together on the same thing. Collaboration is an important relationship skill that can sometimes be tricky but really pays off in the long run! Let's give this some practice with a fun art activity by working with someone else on ONE drawing. Remember this activity is about working together. You might feel frustrated by what your partner draws, but that's part of the challenge! Have fun seeing what you can create together!

Materials:

- Journal or paper
- Drawing tools (crayons, colored pencils and/or markers)

Steps:

1. Find a partner or "collaborator."
2. Each person will use a different color drawing tool.
3. Decide who will start the collaborative drawing first.
4. The first draw-er begins by making a mark on the page. The next draw-er will add their mark. It's up to each person what they draw each time—it could be a line, shape or symbol.
5. Repeat this process back and forth, taking turns. This activity will require patience and communication—two great skills for collaborators!
6. Make two drawings so you can each get a turn making the first mark.

Big picture questions:

1. Think about your process. What parts did you find easy? Challenging?
2. Think about how you worked together. What worked? What could use more work?
3. How might collaboration be helpful at school? In your community?
4. Where do you see others in your community collaborating?

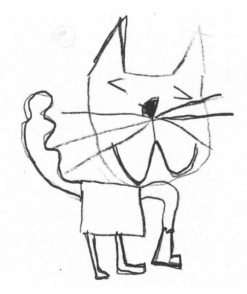

Student example

FOLLOW THE SCRIBBLER

Taking turns leading and following is important in building healthy relationships. Let's play a game where we take turns leading and following. How do you feel when you are leading? How do you feel when you are following?

Materials:

- Journal or paper
- Drawing tools (crayons, colored pencils and/or markers)

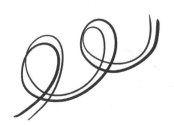

Steps:

1. Get into pairs, select a drawing tool and decide who will be the leader and who will be the follower.
2. The leader will place their drawing tool on the paper and the follower will place their drawing tool next to the leader's.
3. The leader will move their drawing tool around the paper and the follower will follow.
4. See what it feels like to go fast or slow. After 1–2 minutes, switch!
5. Extra points! Work together to see if you can turn your scribble into something!

Big picture questions:

1. Think about your process. What parts did you find fun? What parts were challenging?
2. What parts do you like about being a leader? A follower?
3. Think about your relationships with friends and family. How do you decide who is the leader and who is the follower? Is it always the same?

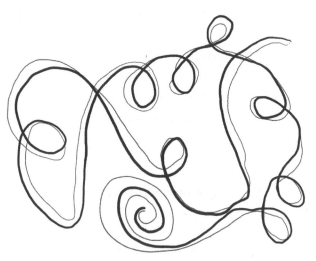

Student example

SCRIBBLE SOLVER

More fun with lines and scribbles! Here's a fun drawing game that helps us practice teamwork and collaborative problem-solving—two very important skills in relationship building!

Materials:

- Journal or paper
- Drawing tools (crayons, colored pencils and/or markers)

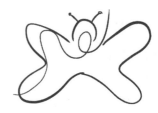

Steps:

1. Find a partner, select a drawing tool and decide who will be the scribbler and who will be the solver.
2. The scribbler will place their drawing tool on the paper and the solver will say "go!"
3. When the solver feels ready, they will say "stop!" and the scribbler will stop.
4. The scribbler and the solver will work together to find an image in the scribble.
5. Feel free to turn the drawing around and look at it from all sides.
6. Once an image is found, the solver will use a different color and add lines and shapes to bring out the image.
7. Now switch! Scribbler becomes the solver and the solver the scribbler!

Big picture questions:

1. When might it be fun to play this game? Who would you play with?
2. Did you and your partner see different images in the scribble? How did you decide which image to bring out?
3. Take a few turns so that you have more than two images. Can you organize the images to create a story?

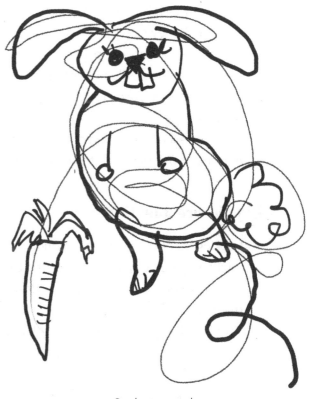

Student example

BLIND CONTOUR PARTNER PORTRAIT

Building and taking care of relationships is fun but also can take time and effort. Working to really see and understand our friends, families and classmates is important in creating healthy relationships. Let's practice this by playing a fun game that has us look carefully at our partner and take turns creating blind contour portraits!

Materials:

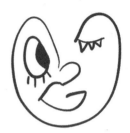

- Journal or paper
- Drawing tools (crayons, colored pencils and/or markers)
- (Optional: watercolor paints, brushes and water)

Steps:

1. Find a partner, select a drawing tool and decide which partner will be the draw-er and which will be the poser.
2. The draw-er will place their drawing tool on the paper and looking very carefully at their partner/ poser, draw all the different lines and shapes (or contours) they see in their partner's face. Be sure to not look at your paper or lift your drawing tool! It will look silly and that's part of the fun!
3. Now switch! The draw-er becomes the poser and the poser the draw-er.
4. After you each have a blind contour portrait, use drawing or painting tools to color in the spaces.

Big picture questions:

1. Looking slowly and carefully at another person might not be something we do all the time. Describe your experience as the draw-er? As the poser?
2. Take a look at your image. What colors did you choose and why? How do they represent the poser?
3. Take a look at the image of you made by your partner. How do you feel looking at the image?

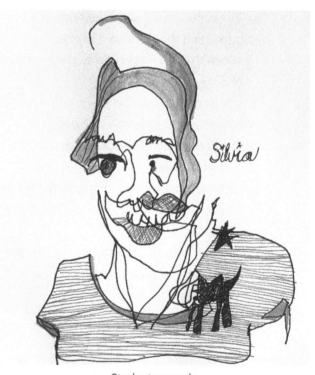

Student example

WHEN THE WINNER IS WE...THE WINNER IS ME!

Celebrating our personal and collective strengths is a great skill for developing relationships! A lot of the time the things that we enjoy doing are also the things that we are good at. It feels good to have others notice and appreciate the things that we are good at. Let's explore and celebrate some of our and our classmates' skills and talents!

Materials:

- Journal or paper
- Drawing tools (crayons, colored pencils and/or markers)

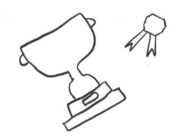

Steps:

1. Begin by thinking of, discussing or listing all the things you enjoy doing.
2. Of all those things that you enjoy doing, what do you feel good at? Being a good friend? Making cupcakes? Or maybe playing with your little cousins?
3. In your journal or on a piece of paper, do your best to draw a prize ribbon or a trophy shape.
4. Fill your shape with words, images, lines, shapes or color to represent your unique skills or talents.
5. If comfortable, share with a classmate or class, or hang awards in the classroom for all to share! Celebrate the similarities and the differences!

Big picture questions:

1. How did it feel to celebrate your personal skills and talents? Your classmates' skills and talents?
2. Sometimes people might say it's not good to say you are good at something, that it is "bragging." What do you think? Are there times when it's helpful and important to celebrate what you're good at? What's the difference?

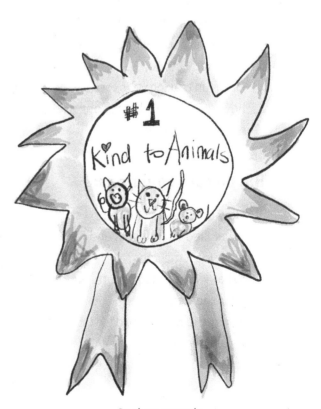

Student example

MY THEME SONG

A "theme song" is usually played at the beginning of a show or movie and sets us up to know what the show will be like. We just learned about how when The Winner Is We… The Winner Is Me! Let's make our own theme song that represents our friends or our class! Would the theme song be fast, silly, loud, quiet?

Materials:

- Journal or paper
- Any mark-making tools

Steps:

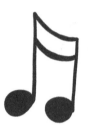

1. You and your group can make up your own tune for this activity but if you would like a little extra support, think of a song you already know. You can change the lyrics!
2. Once you and your group have selected your song, start to add/change the words while keeping the same melody.
3. Write down the words to your song and decorate your paper with bright colors that put you in a happy mood.
4. Have fun making your very own theme song, and hey, maybe your theme song needs some dance moves to go with it!

Big picture questions:

1. How does your theme song sound out loud?
2. What kind of thoughts and feelings do you hear in your theme song?
3. What kind of instruments would you need for your theme song?
4. If your theme song had a dance to go with it, how would it look?

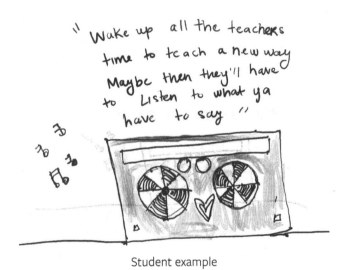

Student example

Chapter 5

RESPONSIBLE DECISION-MAKING

"From my perspective, hearing the students ask for more workshops was definitely a sign that they were gaining something from what we were offering. During the last workshop, some students expressed sadness when they learned that it would be our last meeting. During these same workshops, many students expressed how proud they felt after creating their own SEL video, a tool that they shared with other students as well. In general, I feel that these art workshops offered the students new and creative ways to approach everyday challenges through a combination of art-making and mindfulness exercises."

ART THERAPIST TRAINEE STATEMENT ABOUT FACILITATING CLASSROOM SEL DROP-INS

This quote was gathered from a graduate student trainee who participated in summer SEL workshops offered to students at the height of the COVID-19 pandemic. In this workshop middle school students were being asked to reflect on their creative coping skills in order to co-create instructional art videos aimed at improving community wellness. The videos centered on teaching others how to use art and mindfulness as a healthy coping skill to address low mood and helplessness about the stay-at-home orders. Mentorship and a sense of belonging within the group carried them throughout the task to think critically about how to address mental health needs of young people their age. Offering a new and challenging art experience was a great opportunity to practice cooperation and persistence.

Responsible decision-making highlights for students that they can make meaningful choices for themselves that can also have an impact on their community. Self-awareness and social awareness lead up to the more thoughtful evaluations. Exploring responsible decision-making guides them to make safe choices that evaluate the impact of actions. As educators this is all we hope for, that the critical thinking skills we offer now will help our students make an impact in this world.

Offering opportunities to discuss responsible choices can contribute to balance and harmony in your classroom. A space where students can use curiosity and an open mind when presented with a problem. This might look like a calm and reflective opportunity to pause and think about what they value personally and how it compares to values of the classroom, school culture and community at large. It can offer a sense of agency, empowerment and safety to stand up for others and matters of social justice.

Talking about a shared value for your classroom can be enhanced when we offer art experiences that help students imagine and create a visual reference to these values. It offers the space necessary to deepen an understanding of how their behavior has an impact on society at large. For example, "what does a safe classroom look like" can be expanded further to explore what all humans need to feel safe. Using the art to think critically about this topic brings up important universal questions about what is socially acceptable behavior for a just world. The art process can give students an opportunity to think more about problems they might experience in their lives and safe ways to explore consequences of their actions. Art activities allow students to apply skills such as imagination, creativity, teamwork and collaboration—all useful tools that can be applied to real world situations!

Creating opportunities to partner students together when creating the art can facilitate brainstorming, analyzing and coming to a group consensus. When it's time to share the art reflections, consider having the students share in small groups so that they can see the different ways students were able to come up with creative solutions.

TOUCHSTONES

A touchstone is a great tool to help guide us in making good personal decisions. A touchstone can represent our values, beliefs and things that we always come back to when faced with a challenge. What are things that are important to you? When you are faced with a difficult decision what do you come back to?

Materials:

- Journal or paper
- Colored pencils or crayons, or watercolor paint palette, brushes, water
- (Optional: watercolor paper)

Steps:

1. Think about the last time you had to make a tough decision. How did you help yourself? Discuss as a class, with a person sitting close by and/or write your thoughts in your journal.
2. Draw a stone shape on your paper or in your journal.
3. Decorate the stone shape with words, colors, shapes, symbols that represent what you came back to when faced with a difficult decision.
4. Share with your class or with someone sitting close to you.

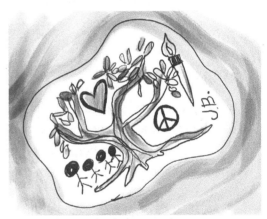

Student example

Big picture questions:

1. Take a look at your image. What do some of the lines, shapes, colors and symbols represent to you?
2. Take a look at your classmates' images. Are there any similarities in the values and beliefs you chose to represent?
3. Think about the values and beliefs you chose to represent. Do you remember when these values and beliefs became important? Where did these values and beliefs come from?

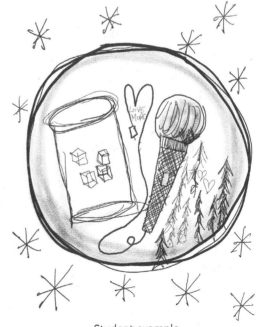

Student example

"OWNING IT"

Have you ever made a choice that was not the most, let's say, thoughtful? Maybe you teased someone a little too much and accidentally hurt their feelings? Or perhaps you took something that wasn't yours? Did you feel bad about it? Likely the answer to these questions we just asked is "yes." Being able to say we did something wrong and "owning it" can be really hard. Being able to "own it" and take responsibility for our actions is a great skill in life. We aren't our mistakes. It's what we do about the mistake that shows who we are. No one is perfect and we all make mistakes. Taking responsibility and understanding our feelings helps us grow.

Materials:

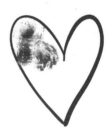

- Journal or paper
- Colored pencils or crayons, or watercolor paint palette, brushes, water

Steps:

1. Think of the last time you did something that you can take ownership of. Perhaps you used unkind words with your brother, or you were jealous of a friend and said or did something you felt bad about.
2. Think about the feelings you felt in your heart when that happened.
3. Use watercolor and/or paint to demonstrate those feelings using lines, shape and color.
4. Perhaps this will help you the next time you want to express your feelings and "own it" when you make a mistake.

Big picture questions:

1. Take a look at your image. What types of feelings do you see or were you trying to show in your art piece?
2. When a friend or family member makes a mistake (hurts your feelings or breaks something special) what can they say or do to show you that they are "owning it" or taking responsibility for their actions?

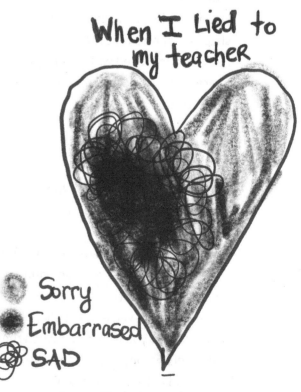

Student example

CHOOSE YOUR OWN PATH

Our days are filled with lots of choices and times when we must make decisions. Making a decision can feel stressful or hard sometimes because we might worry that it's not the *right* decision. However, if we listen to our bodies, thoughts and feelings we might see that oftentimes there are many ways to get to the same place. Let's practice exploring how there are lots of choices, decisions or pathways that can lead to the same destination.

Materials:

- Journal or paper
- Drawing tools (crayons, colored pencils and/or markers)

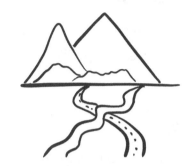

Steps:

1. In your journal or on a piece of paper, do your best to draw a line from one side of your paper to the other. This will be your "horizon line."
2. On this "horizon line" create an image that represents a place or destination where you would like to go.
3. Beginning at the bottom of your page, create multiple pathways (or choices) that lead to your destination, i.e. roads, tracks, etc.
4. Add images that show what you might encounter on each pathway.
5. Share as a class or with someone close to you.

Big picture questions:

1. What are some choices you have had to make recently?
2. Are there certain choices you find more difficult to make than others? Easier than others?
3. What are the different strategies you use when making a decision?

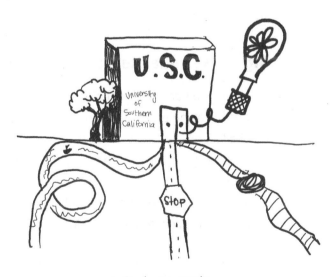

Student example

89

FINDING A RESILIENT VOICE

When things get hard or you have to make tough decisions, there can often be a little voice in your head that will encourage you to keep going. Being resilient is being able to keep going or bounce back during challenges. Resilient folks have a way of talking themselves through hard stuff. Let's give you a chance to practice. Can you think of a phrase that helps you get through something hard?

Materials:

- Journal or paper
- Drawing tools (crayons, colored pencils and/or markers)

Steps:

1. Use your journal to create a scenario about a character finding their resilient voice.
2. On the first page, draw a character who is having a hard day. Draw thought bubbles to explore how their thoughts are making them feel down.
3. On the next page. Draw the same character, only this time ... they have brought more resilient thoughts into their mind, changing their day around.

Big picture questions:

1. What are some resilient thoughts you discovered that helped your character during their challenge?
2. How do the thoughts change your character's actions?
3. Think of a time when you felt challenged. What types of resilient thoughts could you think about?

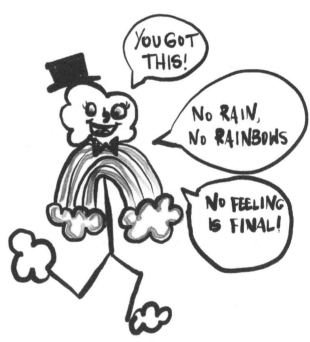

Student example

UPSTANDER EXPLORATION

An upstander is someone who stands up for others. An upstander doesn't just sit back and watch while someone is being mistreated, they speak up and speak out in safe ways so that unkind behavior stops. Let's see if we can play out a little scenario so that we can practice this skill with art.

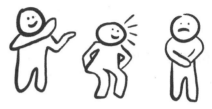

Materials:

- Journal or paper
- Any mark-making tools

Steps:

1. Take your journal and split the paper in half with a big line down the middle. If you want more space to tell your story, you can break your page into four parts by putting a cross on your paper.
2. On the right side of the page, draw a picture of some "not so nice" behavior that happens at school.
3. On the left side of the page, draw a picture of yourself coming in as the upstander to put a stop to the situation.
4. Think about what you might say or do in that situation using speech bubbles or thought bubbles.
5. Show the person next to you and see what they think.

Big picture questions:

1. Being an upstander can bring up a lot of feelings. What types of feelings do you think might come up when you act as an "upstander"?
2. What things make it hard to be an upstander? What are things that make it easier?
3. What types of school rules and agreements make it easier to be an upstander?

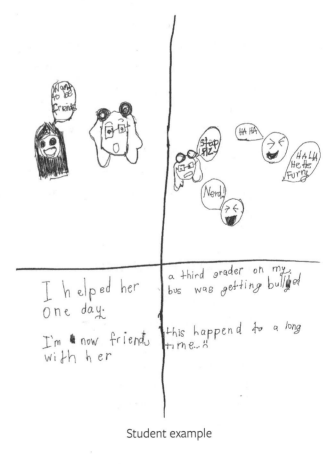

Student example

RANDOM ACT OF KINDNESS

We don't need a reason to be kind. Being kind can really make someone's day. When someone is kind to you, how does it make you feel? How do you feel when you are kind to someone else? Showing a little bit of kindness to someone, even if there's no special reason, helps let them know that they are appreciated in the community. In this activity, you will make little tokens of kindness that you can offer to someone unexpectedly.

Materials:

- Journal or paper
- Drawing tools (crayons, colored pencils and/or markers)
- (Optional: something sturdy for your base, e.g. cardstock/recycled cardboard, paint and brushes, decorative flair such as glitter, beads etc., scissors and glue)

Steps:

1. Start thinking about people in your life who could use a random act of kindness from you.
2. Draw or use your scissors to create shapes for your gift. It can be hearts, circles, stars—whatever you want.
3. Use art materials to add happy colors that will brighten someone's day.
4. Have fun handing out your gift or leaving your gift as a little surprise that will make someone's day.

Big picture questions:

1. Who did you choose to share a random act of kindness with? How did you make this choice?
2. How did you feel when you were creating your random act of kindness? And when you were handing them out?
3. What are other ways we can show community members we appreciate them?

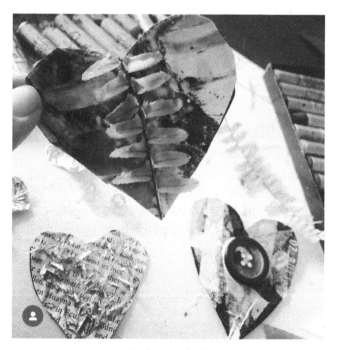

Student example

R-E-S-P-E-C-T (PLACE AND THINGS)

Showing respect isn't just about honoring and listening to the needs and feelings of others. We can also show respect for places and things too. Remember, respect is about demonstrating you care. Let's think about our classroom. Look around you, are there things in the classroom that you can show respect to? You bet. It's part of our school culture to take good care of our learning space. Let's think about things we can show respect for at school by making a spider map.

Materials:

- Journal or paper
- Any mark-making tools

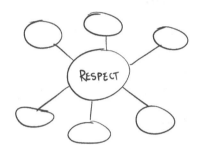

Steps:

1. Brainstorm with your class all the ways we can show things respect in our classroom by making a spider map like the one pictured here.
2. Next draw examples of how that might look in your classroom.
3. You can make your own spider map, or you and your class can make a huge spider map for your classroom wall so you can all remember how to demonstrate respect at school.
4. If you finish quickly, draw a picture of your classroom.

Big picture questions:

1. Let's look at other drawings, do you see similarities?
2. Why do we need to take care of our things at our school?

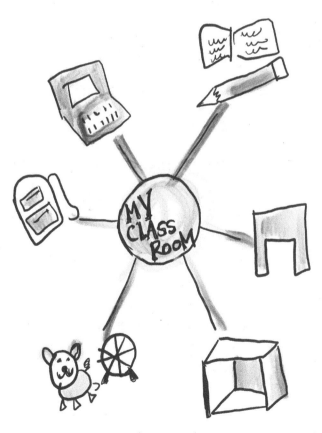

Student example

WE MUST PERSIST!

Sometimes you just have to keep going because it can take a bunch of tries and lots of setbacks to achieve your goals—kind of like climbing a mountain. Do you have a "mountain" you are climbing? Is there anything hard in your life? In this exercise you will draw a time in your life when you have had to persist and keep going, or at least you had a plan to try. What is your personal "mountain"?

Materials:

- Journal or paper
- Drawing tools (crayons, colored pencils and/or markers)

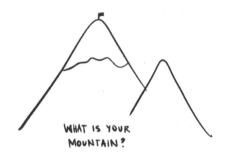

Steps:

1. Use your drawing tools to draw yourself on the big "mountain" that you are climbing.
2. If you can't think of an example, you can make a story about someone else climbing the mountain and overcoming a challenging task.
3. Think about all the things that can help you get through it, for example, friends and family, deep breaths, asking for help, eating healthy, getting enough rest, positive thinking...

Big picture questions:

1. We are using a mountain as a symbol for getting through a challenge. Why do we use a mountain as a symbol? What are the things we need if we are actually climbing a mountain? For example, planning, equipment, time and helpers?
2. In what way is climbing a mountain similar to getting through something very difficult? Do we also need planning, equipment, time and helpers? In what way?

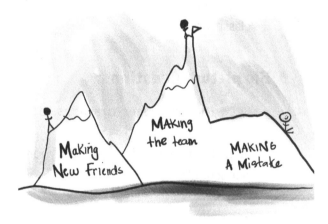

Student example

"KEEP AT IT" BACKPACK

When you climb a "mountain" you need certain tools with you in your backpack. When you are trying to get through something hard in life you need tools too. "Keep at it" tools are the things that help you keep your body calm and make good decisions for you and those around you. You probably know a lot of ways to keep your body calm already. What objects or items help motivate you for hard things?

Materials:

- Journal or paper
- Drawing tools (crayons, colored pencils and/or markers)

Steps:

1. In your journal, imagine what you need for your "keep at it" backpack. For example, a fidget spinner or something that smells nice and calming. What helps you when you get through hard things? Something soft to hold in your hand?

2. Use your drawing materials to do your best to draw a backpack.

3. Fill up your backpack with all of the things that help you stay calm. Perhaps you have a picture of your best friend who always reminds you to keep trying?

4. Share as a class or with someone close to you. What are their tools? Could you add these tools to your backpack?

Big picture questions:

1. How does our "keep at it" backpack help us with personal wellness?

2. When might you use what is inside your backpack?

3. Do you have something that is calming for each of your five senses? Share with the group similarities and differences.

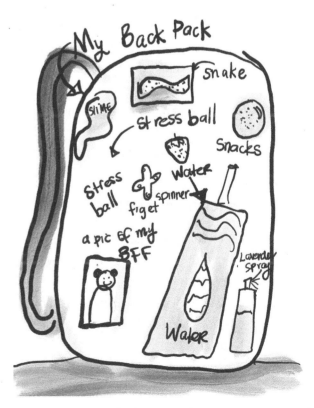

Student example

SOLUTION MACHINE

Creating solutions to problems takes imagination, creativity, teamwork and collaboration! Many of the world's problems have been solved by groups of creative problem-solvers. Let's work together and use our imagination to create solution machines!

Materials:

- Journal or paper
- Drawing tools (crayons, colored pencils and/or markers)
- (Optional: recyclables, found objects, magazine collage, glue sticks)

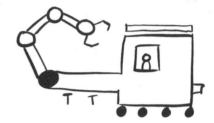

Steps:

1. Create a group with one or more of your classmates.
2. Work together to decide on a school, community or world problem that you would like to explore solutions for.
3. Brainstorm together all the different ways that you might solve this problem—be as imaginative and creative as you can!
4. Work together to draw or construct an image or sculpture of a machine that might be a solution to the problem.
5. Share with your classmates!

Big picture questions:

1. Were there any disagreements when you created your solution machine? How did you work through them?
2. Wow, it looks like you were all thinking outside the box. When in life do you think it's important to do that?

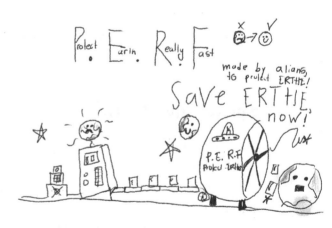

Student example

WHAT DO CITIES NEED TO THRIVE?

Let's use the art process to create an imagined city where everybody has their needs met. What do we need for cities to thrive? What types of spaces are important for people to be happy? A museum where we can be inspired by beautiful art? A public garden for healthy food to eat? A gathering space where folks can come together to celebrate? What will your city look like?

Materials:

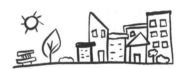

- Journal or paper
- Drawing tools (crayons, colored pencils and/or markers)
- (Optional: colored paper, scissors and glue)

Steps:

1. Brainstorm with your class some ideas about what your city might hold.
2. Using your art materials, start mapping out what your city might look like. Put a sign on your building so we know what it's used for.
3. Have fun using your imagination.
4. When everyone is all done, line all of your cities up to make a super-duper city.

Big picture questions:

1. What will you name your city?
2. Who lives in your city? What is important to the people who live in your city?
3. How does it feel to see your buildings come together to form a city?

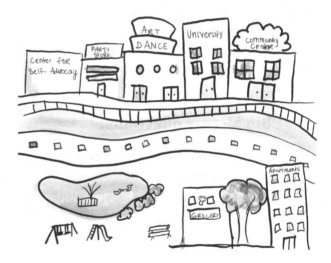

Student example

WHAT DO YOU HAVE TO SAY?

Thinking about others is important for creating a safe and just (fair) world. Empathy (thinking about how others feel) and kindness can connect us in wonderful ways. This world is so big and there are so many people here. If you could say anything to the whole world, what would you say?

Materials:

- Journal or paper
- Drawing tools (crayons, colored pencils and/or markers)

Steps:

1. Use your drawing tools to make a globe shape.
2. Think of some wishes you might want for others so that they can feel safe and loved.
3. Use your materials to draw your message to others.
4. Share your message with the class or with someone close to you.
5. Post your art in your school community for others to see!

Big picture questions:

1. Do you think one person can impact the whole world? Why?
2. What happens when you find other people who feel exactly how you do?

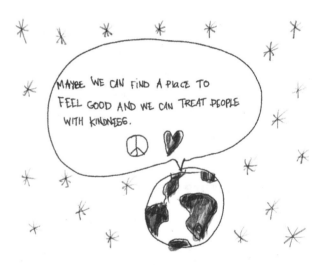

Student example

Author Biographies

Dr. Jessica Bianchi, LMFT, ATR-BC. Born to a children's book author/illustrator and a social worker, it seems natural that Jessica would become an art therapist. Before discovering art therapy, Jessica began her career as an elementary school teacher. Jessica used her art-making to teach every subject—from Math to Social Studies. Additionally, Jessica used art making as a means to connect with her students. Seeing the power of art to support social, emotional and academic growth, Jessica pursued a Masters in Art Therapy and later a Doctorate in Education for Social Justice—focusing on how therapeutic art-making might increase students' resilience and protective factors for adversity later in life. Jessica worked for ten years in community mental health with adolescents and families. Currently, Jessica lives in Los Angeles with her family and is a professor at Loyola Marymount University in the Department of Marital and Family Therapy with Specialized Training in Art Therapy, and the Director of the Department's Helen B. Landgarten Art Therapy Clinic.

Amber Cromwell, LMFT ATR-BC. First and foremost, Amber sees herself as an artist. It wasn't until later in life that she realized she had been practicing her own version of art for SEL well before she chose art education as her area of focus during her undergraduate studies. Her path as an artist and educator eventually led to the "aha moment" when she discovered the field of art therapy. She has had the honor to work with young people of all ages and abilities, families and adults within a variety of settings, including Los Angeles and surrounding area school districts, community outpatient centers within the Department of Mental Health, Cedars Sinai Medical Center, Loyola Marymount University Helen B. Landgarten Art Therapy Clinic, residential care for adolescents and families, programs for incarcerated individuals and a host of non-profit organizations. All of these have affirmed an alliance towards a social justice perspective, a passion to utilize art as a means to equity and a mission to champion a community approach to mental health.

References

ATCB (2024). *What Is Art Therapy?* ATCB. Accessed on 04/14/24 at www.atcb.org/what-is-art-therapy.

Bath, H. (2015). The three pillars of traumawise care: Healing in the other 23 hours. *Reclaiming Children & Youth, 23*(4).

Brunzell, T., Stokes, H. & Waters, L. (2016). Trauma-informed positive education: Using positive psychology to strengthen vulnerable students. *Contemporary School Psychology, 20*(1), 63–83.

CASEL (2022). *SEL Policy at the State Level: A Systemic Approach Can Align State Policies, Resources, and Actions to Support SEL.* CASEL. Accessed on 03/14/24 at https://casel.org/systemic-implementation/sel-policy-at-the-state-level/#CA.

CASEL (2024). *What Is SEL?* CASEL. Accessed on 03/14/24 at https://drc.casel.org/what-is-sel.

Dissanayake, E. (1995). *Homo Aestheticus: Where Art Comes from and Why?* Seattle, WA: University of Washington Press.

Gregory, D.C. (2002) *The Stages of Artistic Development.* Southwest Texas State University. Summarized from V. Lowenfeld (1987) *Creative and Mental Growth (3rd ed.)* Hoboken, NJ: Prentice Hall. Available at: https://static1.squarespace.com/static/64fa67d6edfa144faeac4557/t/6608b550eebbb645f671f388/1711846736994/stages_of_art_development-1.pdf

Little Hoover Commission (2021). *Children's Mental Health: Addressing the Impact.* Accessed on 04/14/24 at www.lhc.ca.gov/report/covid-19-and-childrens-mental-health-addressing-impact.

Ray, C.D. (ed.) (2016). *A Therapist's Guide to Child Development: The Extraordinarily Normal Years.* New York: Taylor & Francis.

Rubin, J. (1978). *Child Art Therapy: Understanding and Helping Children Grow Through Art.* New York: Van Nostrand Reinhold.

Wigelsworth, M., Verity, L., Mason, C., Qualter, P. & Humphrey, N. (2022). Social and emotional learning in primary schools: A review of the current state of evidence. *British Journal of Educational Psychology, 92*(3), 898–924.

Further Reading

Buchanan, R., Gueldner, B., Tran, K.O. & Merrell, K. (2009). Social and emotional learning in class-rooms: A survey of teachers' knowledge, perceptions, and practices. *Journal of Applied School Psychology, 25*(2), 187–203.

Farrington, C.A., Wright, L., Weiss, E.M., Shewfelt, S. *et al.* (2019). (rep.). *Arts Education and Social-Emotional Learning Outcomes among K-12 Students: Developing a Theory of Action* (pp. 1–48). Chicago, IL: University of Chicago Consortium on School Research.

Ghahramani, N., Khakpour, M., Ahadi, H. & Shabani, M. (2021). The effectiveness of visual arts therapy on self-expression and self-esteem of women with mental disorders. *Iranian Journal of Psychiatry, 16*(1), 1-7.

Gruber, H. & Oepen, R. (2018). Emotion regulation strategies and effects in art-making: A narrative synthesis. *The Arts in Psychotherapy, 59*, 65–74.

Merrell, K.W. & Gueldner, B.A. (2010) *Social and Emotional Learning in the Classroom Promoting Mental Health and Academic Success* (pp.48–66). *New York:* Guilford Publications.

Zakaria, M.Z., Yunus, F. & Mohamed, S. (2021). Drawing activities enhance preschoolers socio emotional development. *Southeast Asia Early Childhood, 10*(1), 18–27.